.ent
for Cervical Spondylosis
Using Massage

of related interest

Illustrated Treatment for Migraine using Acupuncture, Moxibustion and Tuina Massage
Cui Chengbin and Xing Xiaomin
ISBN 978 1 84819 061 0

Tuina/ Massage Manipulations
Basic Principles and Techniques
Chief Editor: Li Jiangshan
ISBN 978 1 84819 058 0

Needling Techniques for Acupuncturists
Basic Principles and Techniques
Chief Editor: Professor Chang Xiaorong
ISBN 978 1 84819 057 3

Basic Theories of Traditional Chinese Medicine
Edited by Zhu Bing and Wang Hongcai
Advisor: Cheng Xinnong
ISBN 978 1 84819 038 2

Diagnostics of Traditional Chinese Medicine
Edited by Zhu Bing and Wang Hongcai
Advisor: Cheng Xinnong
ISBN 978 1 84819 036 8

Meridians and Acupoints
Edited by Zhu Bing and Wang Hongcai
Advisor: Cheng Xinnong
ISBN 978 1 84819 037 5

Acupuncture Therapeutics
Edited by Zhu Bing and Wang Hongcai
Advisor: Cheng Xinnong
ISBN 978 1 84819 039 9

Case Studies from the Medical Records of Leading Chinese Acupuncture Experts
Edited by Zhu Bing and Wang Hongcai
Advisor: Cheng Xinnong
ISBN 978 1 84819 046 7

Illustrated Treatment for Cervical Spondylosis Using Massage

Tang Xuezhang and Yu Tianyuan

SINGING
DRAGON

LONDON AND PHILADELPHIA

Editorial Committee: Tang Xuezhang, Yu Tianyuan, Jia
Yunfang, Zheng Huimin, Yuan Zhilin and Wu Fan
Translator: Yang Fan
Photographer: Yu Xiaowen

This edition published in 2011
by Singing Dragon
an imprint of Jessica Kingsley Publishers
in co-operation with People's Military Medical Press
116 Pentonville Road
London N1 9JB, UK
and
400 Market Street, Suite 400
Philadelphia, PA 19106, USA

www.singingdragon.com

First published in 2009
by People's Military Medical Press

Copyright © People's Military Medical Press 2009 and 2011

Library of Congress Cataloging in Publication Data
A CIP catalog record for this book is available from the Library of Congress

British Library Cataloguing in Publication Data
A CIP catalogue record for this book is available from the British Library

ISBN 978 1 84819 062 7

Printed and bound in Great Britain
by the MPG Books Group

Contents

About the Authors

Tang Xuezhang, male, born in 1963, associate chief physician, graduated in acupuncture and Tuina from Shanghai University of Traditional Chinese Medicine. In his more than 20 years of working as a doctor, based on inheriting and carrying forward the traditional medicine of his homeland, he has developed a complete set of manipulation procedures, based on integration of traditional Chinese and Western medicine treatments, and excels in treating conditions such as cervical spondylosis, periarthritis of the shoulder, lumbar disc prolapse, injury of the sacroiliac joint, and myofascitis, using manipulation. He has been invited to Japan, Switzerland, and the Republic of Kazakhstan, to work and exchange experience. He has published more than ten medical professional theses, and has had a part in editing two medical academic books. At present he is the director of the TCM Massage Department of the China–Japan Friendship Hospital, the Ministry of Health. He also works part time as a member of the standing committee of massage of the Beijing Association of Traditional Chinese Medicine. He is a member of the health preserving committee of the Chinese Medical Doctor Association, and a specialist editor of *Chinese Massotherapy Magazine*.

Yu Tianyuan, male, born in 1965, MD, professor, doctorial tutor, graduated in integrated traditional and Western medicine from Beijing University of Chinese Medicine. He works in Beijing University of Chinese Medicine, teaching, researching, and in clinical practice, focusing on Tuina massage, acupuncture, and moxibustion. His book *Tuina Massage* is one of the Beijing Municipal Excellent Teaching Materials. He has been awarded the third prize in the advanced science and technology progress competition at the Science Development Program Awards in Beijing. He has published more than 20 academic books and more than 30 theses.

Preface

Cervical spondylosis manifests in a range of symptoms caused by degeneration of the cervical vertebrae and cervical articulation, involving joint capsules, ligaments, and intervertebral disks, which leads to pathological changes such as instability of the cervical spine, hyperosteogeny, hypertrophy of ligaments, hypertrophy of joint capsules, and calcification, which in turn may stimulate or compress cervical nerve roots, vertebral arteries, the spinal cord, and sympathetic nerves, causing various symptoms. Cervical spondylosis is also called 'cervical degenerative osteoarthritis' or 'cervical syndrome.' Different types of cervical spondylosis can be distinguished according to which tissues are pathologically affected: the stiff neck type of cervical spondylosis; cervical spondylotic radiculopathy; the vertebral artery type of cervical spondylosis; cervical spondylotic myelopathy; sympathetic cervical spondylosis, and a mixed type of cervical spondylosis.

Massage therapy has therapeutic effects, such as relaxing and activating the tendons, regulating tendons and taxis, activating blood circulation to dissipate blood stasis, reducing swelling, and relieving pain by using manipulations on the meridians and acupoints of the human body. Massage therapy is effective for treating traumatological diseases, internal diseases, and pediatric diseases.

Many patients like massage therapy for cervical spondylosis because of its efficacy and painlessness, and it is a major treatment for cervical spondylosis at the present time.

The authors of this book wish to share their clinical experience and hope that after learning what is written in this book and related topics, readers will be able to help patients suffering from cervical spondylosis, and remove their pain.

The editorial committee
Beijing, August 2009

Summary

This book has been written by experienced professors and experts who work in the Tuina Department of Beijing University of Chinese Medicine and in the TCM Massage Department of the China–Japan Friendship Hospital, the Ministry of Health. The book consists of four parts:

1. Introduction to Cervical Spondylosis
2. Fundamentals of Treatment for Cervical Spondylosis
3. Massage Therapy Treatment for Cervical Spondylosis
4. Prevention of Cervical Spondylosis.

The introduction to cervical spondylosis gives a definition of cervical spondylosis and describes pathogeny and corresponding pathogenesis, as well as the clinical manifestations, in detail.

The chapter on treatment fundamentals introduces the essentials regarding meridians and collaterals, acupoints, and basic therapeutic manipulations.

The chapter on massage treatment comprehensively presents the treatment of cervical spondylosis by means of Chinese massage therapy, and also the writers' opinions about misunderstandings of the treatments.

The chapter on preventing cervical spondylosis discusses do's and don'ts that people need to know to take care of their necks, how to do self-massage, and functional exercises for the neck.

This book is a mine of information; both text and illustrations are excellent, and the techniques introduced in the book are practical and described in detail.

It is intended for clinicians, basic medical practitioners, and students in schools of Chinese medicine, as well as for cervical spondylosis patients and their families.

Chapter *1*

Introduction to Cervical Spondylosis

Section I Definition and Presentation

Cervical spondylosis manifests in a range of symptoms caused by degeneration of the cervical vertebrae and cervical articulation, involving joint capsules, ligaments, and intervertebral disks, which leads to pathological changes such as instability of the cervical spine, hyperosteogeny, hypertrophy of ligaments, hypertrophy of joint capsules, and calcification (Figure 1.1a–c, Figure 1.2a–f, Figure 1.3, Figure 1.4), which in turn stimulates or compresses cervical nerve roots, vertebral arteries, the spinal cord, and sympathetic nerves, causing various symptoms. Cervical spondylosis is also called 'cervical degenerative osteoarthritis' or 'cervical syndrome.'

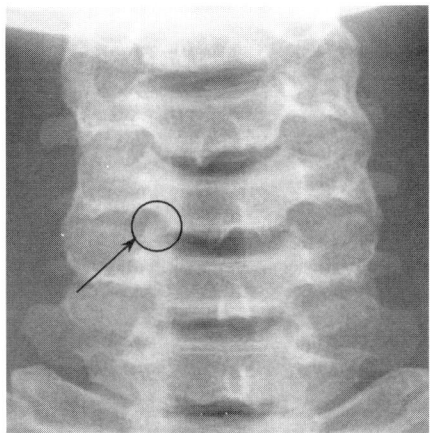

Figure 1.1 Anterior-posterior X-ray view of cervical spine

a. Hyperosteogeny of an uncovertebral joint

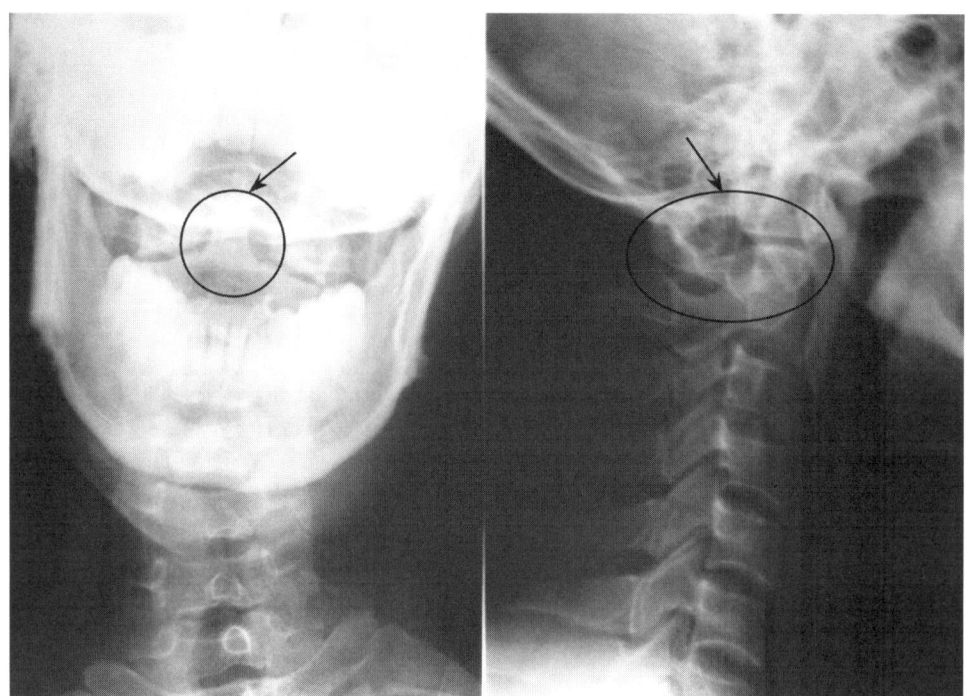

b. Atlanto-axial subluxation

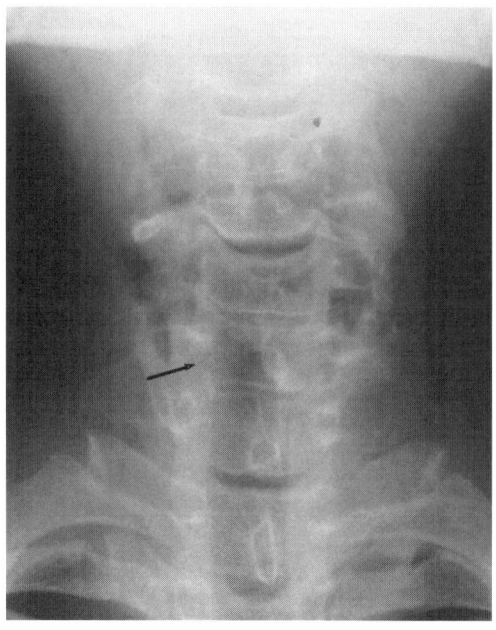

c. Fusion of C6–7

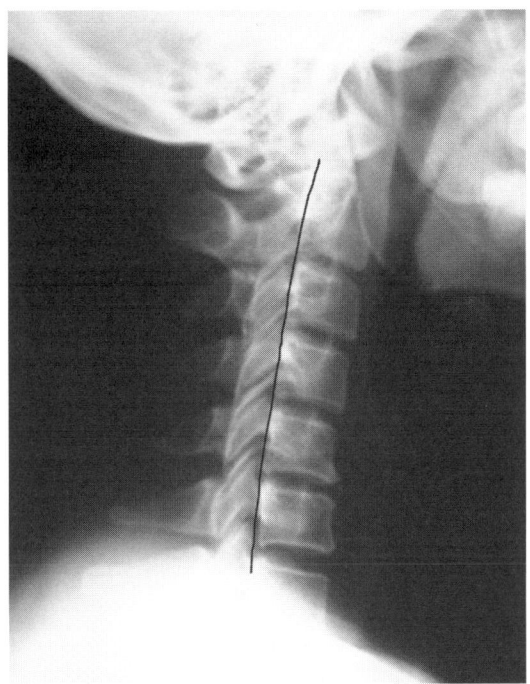

Figure 1.2 Lateral X-ray view of cervical spine

a. Loss of curve of the cervical spine

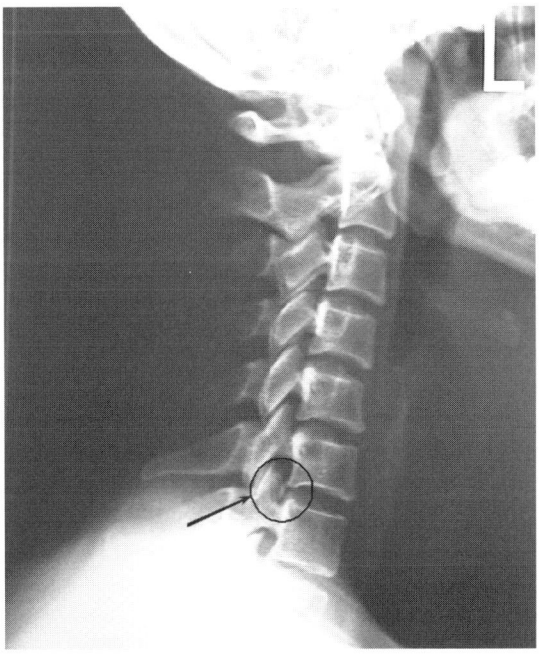

*b. Loss of curve of the cervical spine, with
calcification of the posterior longitudinal ligament*

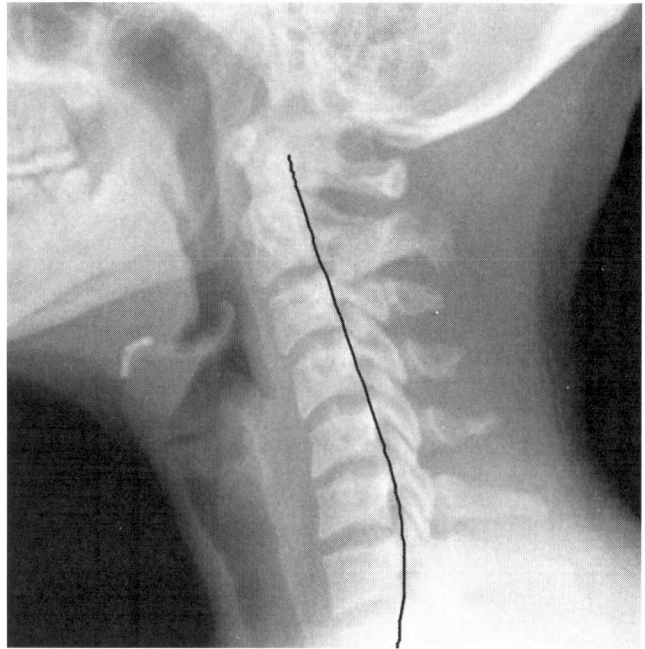

c. Reverse cervical curve

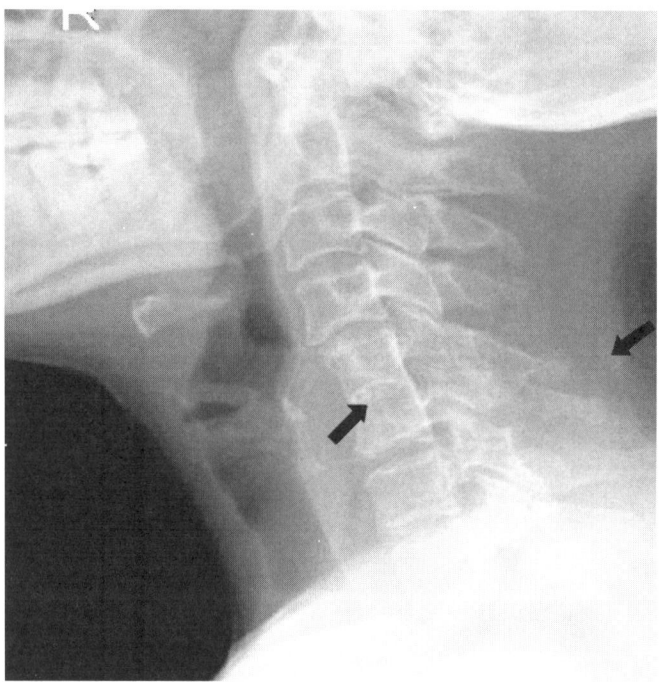

d. Fusion of C5–6 and calcification of ligament of nape

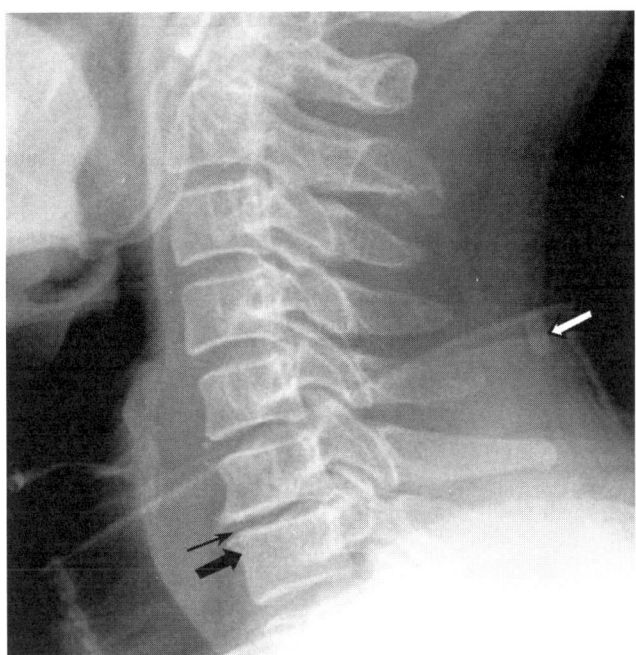

e. Narrowing of C6–7 intervertebral disk space (↑); anterior border hyperosteogeny of cervical vertebrae (↑); calcification of ligament of nape (⇧)

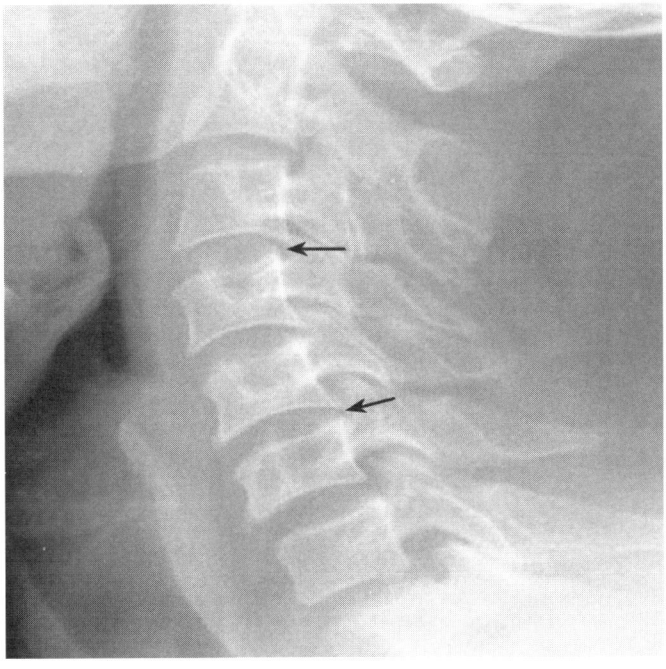

f. Disruption of the line joining the posterior borders of cervical vertebrae

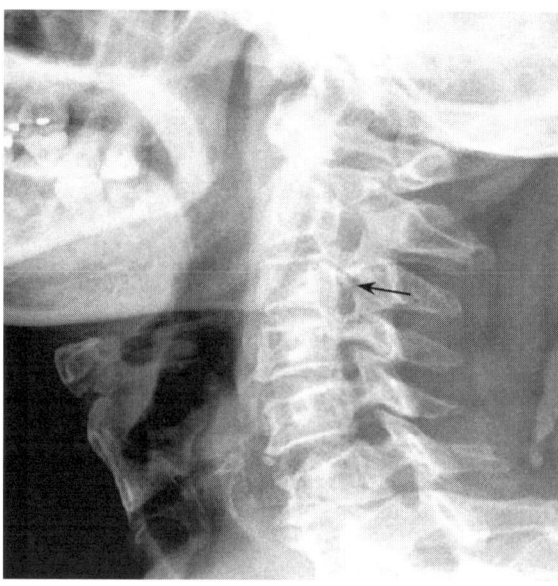

Figure 1.3 Oblique X-ray view of the cervical spine

a. Distortion of cervical intervertebral foramen

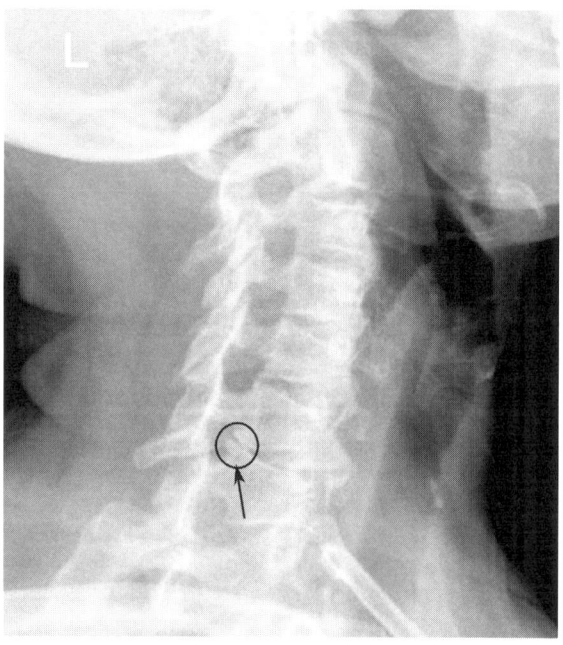

b. Stenosis of intervertebral foramen, hyperosteogeny of uncovertebral joint

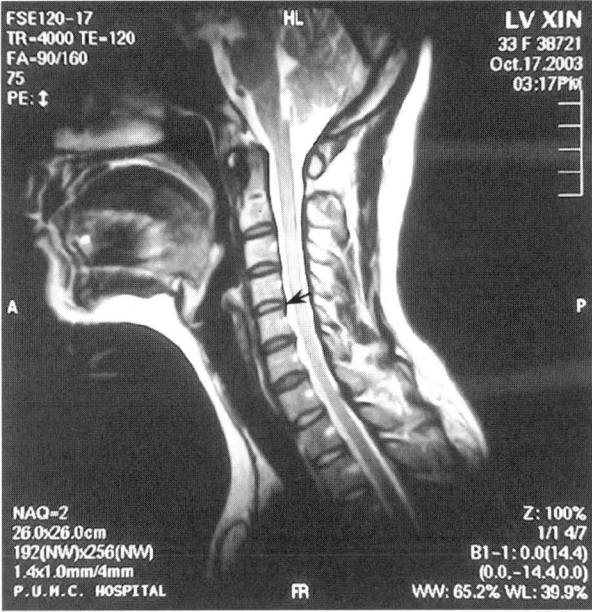

*Figure 1.4 MRI of the cervical spine, showing prolapse
of the C4–5 intervertebral disc*

Different types of cervical spondylosis can be distinguished according to which tissues are pathologically affected:

- the stiff neck type of cervical spondylosis
- cervical spondylotic radiculopathy
- the vertebral artery type of cervical spondylosis
- cervical spondylotic myelopathy
- sympathetic cervical spondylosis
- mixed type of cervical spondylosis.

The *stiff neck type* of cervical spondylosis, also called cervical vertebrae syndrome, mainly affects the nerve roots C1–C4. The main symptoms are neck pain and shoulder pain. Sometimes it is difficult to clearly differentiate the stiff neck type of cervical spondylosis from cervical spondylotic radiculopathy.

Cervical spondylotic radiculopathy is the most common type of all. It mainly affects one side, sometimes both sides. The main symptoms are neck pain and upper limb pain. Sixty percent of cervical spondylosis patients have cervical spondylotic radiculopathy.

The main symptoms of the *vertebral artery type* of cervical spondylosis are vertigo and dizziness. Twenty percent of cervical spondylosis is of this type.

The main symptoms of *cervical spondylotic myelopathy* are sensory disturbance and dyskinesia. Sensory disturbance and dyskinesia begin in the upper limbs and progress to the lower limbs. Twenty percent of cervical spondylosis patients have cervical spondylotic myelopathy. The cause of cervical spondylotic myelopathy in some patients is neck trauma.

The main clinical manifestations of *sympathetic cervical spondylosis* are sympathetic nerve functional disturbance, and parasympathetic nerve functional disturbance. In 10–20 percent of cases, cervical spondylosis is sympathetic cervical spondylosis.

Cervical spondylosis manifesting symptoms of two or more types of cervical spondylosis is called the *mixed type of cervical spondylosis*.

Cervical spondylosis is commonly seen among people aged 30–60, and mostly in patients who bend over their desk for long periods of time – for example, in the field of information technology, accounting, graph plotting, teaching, medicine, and design.

Recurrent stiffness of the neck is a forewarning of cervical spondylosis.

Neck health problems in schoolchildren and students give rising cause for concern as a result of the increasing burden of study these days.

Section II Pathogeny and Pathological Mechanisms

Chronic injuries and degeneration

Chronic injury of the cervical region, for example, as a result of bending over a desk over a long period of time, leads to degeneration of the cervical vertebrae. Degeneration of the cervical vertebrae is the foundation upon which cervical spondylosis may develop. Degeneration of the intervertebral disks leads to narrowing of the intervertebral space and slackness in the joint capsules and the anterior and posterior longitudinal ligaments, reducing the stability of the spine and leading to compensatory hyperplasia. Hyperplasia may arise in uncovertebral joints, intervertebral joints, and centra of vertebrae. A range of symptoms can be triggered when hyperplastic parts stimulate or compress nerve roots, vertebral arteries, the spinal cord, or sympathetic nerves. Hyperplastic sclerotin can directly compress cervical nerves and blood vessels; it can also stimulate surrounding tissues, leading to aseptic inflammation such as hyperemia, and swelling. Hyperemia and swelling cause indirect compression, and in turn trigger symptoms. Symptoms caused by aseptic inflammation are more commonly seen than those triggered by hyperplasia.

Acute injuries

Various acute injuries such as wrenching injuries, collision injuries, and whiplash injuries, can cause varying degrees of damage to intervertebral disks, ligaments, and posterior joint capsules, which leads to reduced stability of the spine or dislocation of cervical vertebrae. This in turn may directly or indirectly stimulate or compress nerves and blood vessels, triggering a range of symptoms.

Deformities

Some deformities, such as spina bifida occulta of the cervical spine, autonomous vertebral fusion, hypertrophy of a cervical transverse process, cervical rib, hypogenesis, or absence of the odontoid process, may lead to cervical spondylosis. These deformities modify mechanical interaction between the cervical vertebrae, which may place stress on those vertebrae which are adjacent to the pathological vertebrae, or may increase the range of movement, speeding up the degeneration process.

Cervical spondylosis comes under various categories of TCM, such as blockage syndrome, atrophy syndrome, headache, dizziness, stiffness of the nape, and shoulder and back pain.

Section III Clinical Manifestations

Stiff neck type of cervical spondylosis

The main symptoms are:

- Aching pain in nape, muscle spasm in nape, stiffness in nape.
- Likelihood of headache; sometimes the headache reaches the forehead and circumocular parts.
- Likelihood of recurrent manifestation (stiff neck, atlantoaxial subluxation, etc.).

Cervical spondylotic radiculopathy

The main symptoms are:

- Neck and shoulder discomfort accompanied by upper limb pain or numbness, which is commonly radiated to the fingers. The pain is described as dull, aching, distending, latent, or electro-radiating pain. The above-mentioned symptoms are likely to be increased by tiredness or a stiff neck.

○ **Pathological changes of C4–5:** Compression of nerve root C5; neck and shoulder pain radiates to the wrist without reaching the hand; tenderness points are located beside the spinous processes of C4–5, on supraspinous muscle; sensory dysfunction of the region behind the neck and below the ear, and of the region of the midline of palmaris longus on the forearm.

○ **Pathological changes of C5–6:** Compression of nerve root C6; neck and shoulder pain radiates to forearm and thumb; tenderness points are located beside the spinous processes of C5–6 and on the medial superior part of the scapula; sensory dysfunction of radial side of forearm and thumb; decrease of myodynamia of biceps brachii; decrease (Figure 1.5) of the tendon reflex of biceps brachii.

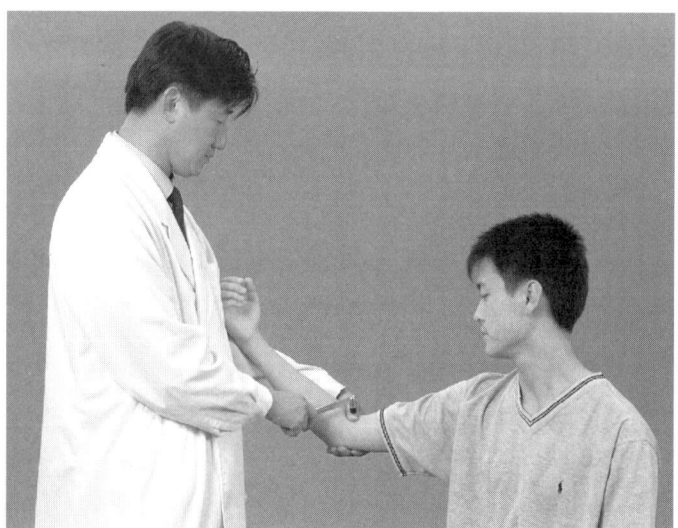

Figure 1.5 Tendon reflex of biceps brachii

○ **Pathological changes of C6–7:** Compression of nerve root C7; neck and shoulder pain radiates to index finger and middle finger; tenderness points are located beside the spinous processes of C6–7 and in the middle part of the region between the scapulae and pectoralis. Decrease of sensory function in the index and middle fingers; decrease of muscle strength of triceps brachii; decrease of tendon reflex (Figure 1.6) of triceps brachii.

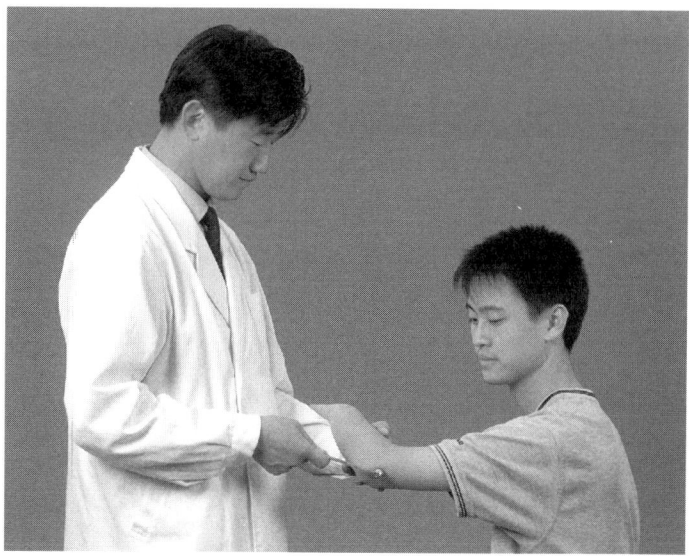

Figure 1.6 Tendon reflex of triceps brachii

- ○ **Pathological changes of C7–T1:** Compression of nerve root C8; neck and shoulder pain radiates to the ring finger and little finger; tenderness points are located on the medial inferior part of the scapula and beside the spinous processes of C7–T1; decrease of sensory function in the little and ring fingers; decrease of handgrip strength; atrophy of skeletal muscles.

- Likelihood of dizziness, carebaria, heaviness and soreness of nape, feelings of heavy load on the back.

- Restricted mobility of nape, deflection of head and neck, spasm of muscles of nape; in the course of time there is a likelihood of muscle atrophy.

- Likelihood of autonomic nerve dysfunction and dysfunction of the nutrient vessel of the autonomic nerve: manifestations are algidity, fever, rash, pallid skin, cyanopathy or swelling of the upper limb, distortion, lustreless nails, a likelihood of fragmentation of nail.

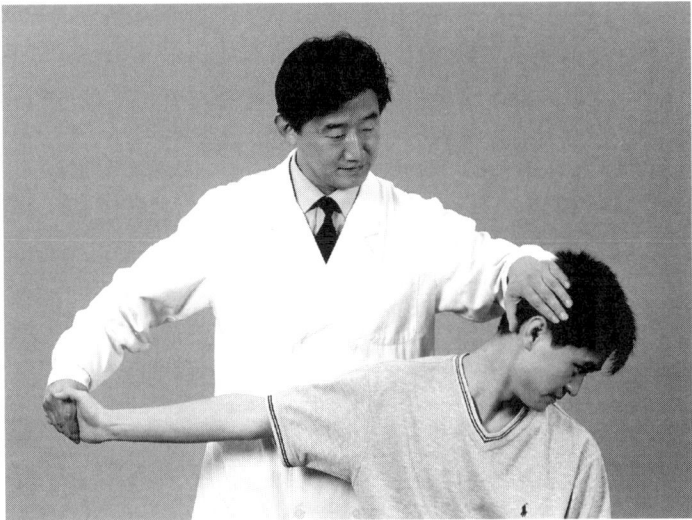

Figure 1.7 Eaton's test

- **Positive sign of Eaton's test** (Figure 1.7): Ask the patient to sit with his head bent slightly forward towards the normal (unaffected) side. The doctor places one hand against the affected side of the patient's head, holding the wrist of the affected side with the other hand. The doctor then stretches in opposite directions with both hands. The positive sign

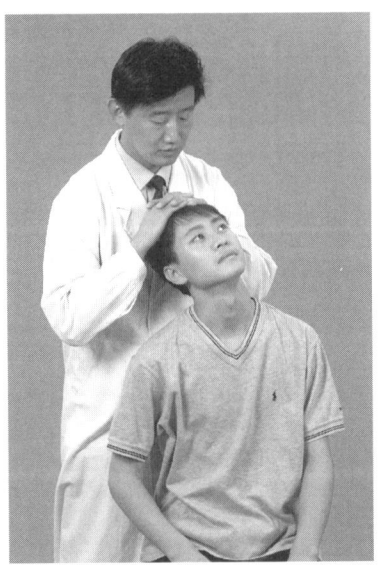 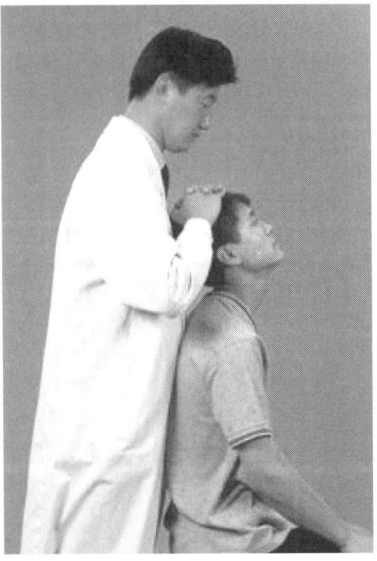

Figure 1.8 Pressure test of the intervertebral foramen

a. Spurling's test   *b. Jackson's test*

is complaint of pain or numbness in the affected upper limb, indicating compression of the brachial plexus.

- **Positive sign of pressure test of the intervertebral foramen** (Figure 1.8): Ask the patient to sit with his head bent backwards and to the side (Spurling's test), or simply bent backwards (Jackson's test). The doctor presses down with both hands on the patient's head. The positive sign of this test is nape pain radiating to the upper limb, indicating compression of the brachial plexus.

Vertebral artery type of cervical spondylosis

The main symptoms are:

- **Cervical vertigo:** A feature of cervical vertigo is positional vertigo when the head is placed in a certain posture. The vertigo is paroxysmal, intermittent, and experienced as rotary, floating, shaky; or as weakness in the lower limb, with unsteadiness when standing, and the illusion of sloping or movement of the ground; always accompanied by symptoms such as tinnitus, diplopia, nystagmus, nausea, and vomiting.

- **Cataplexy:** Likely to occur when moving the head, or with severe vertigo. Falling is caused by sudden numbness and weakness in all four limbs, while fully conscious; most patients are able to get up by themselves.

- **Headache:** The headache is paroxysm; it may last for several minutes, hours, or days. The pain, mainly located on the occiput, calvaria, tempora, is jumping pain or distending pain. Pain radiates to the postauricular region, face, teeth, calvaria, and the ocular region. The cause of the pain is vertebro-basilar artery insufficiency, which leads to dilation of the blood vessels of collateral circulation.

- **Ocular manifestations:** Ocular dysfunction such as blurred vision, diplopia, hallucinatory vision, blindness. A feature of ocular manifestations is that these symptoms are related to the symptoms in the nape: discomfort of the eyes corresponds with motion of the nape.

- **Abnormal sensation:** Likelihood of numbness, acanthesthesia, formication of the face, perioral region, body of the tongue, either in all four limbs or in the limbs and torso of one side of the body, and sensory disturbance of deep sensations.

- **Other:** Likelihood of bulbar paralysis, symptoms implicating the cranial nerves, such as slurred speech, dysphagia, loss of pharyngeal reflex, hoarseness.

- **Check-up:** Likelihood of spasm in the muscles of the nape, tender spots, restricted mobility of the nape, crooked spinous processes.

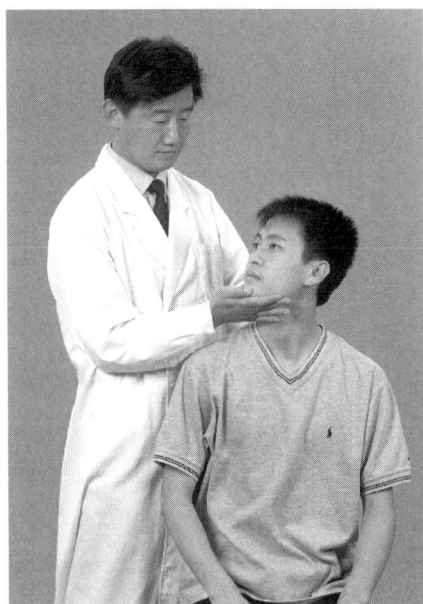

Figure 1.9 Twisting test of vertebral artery

- **Positive sign of twisting test of vertebral artery** (Figure 1.9): Ask the patient to sit and bend his head forwards, backwards, and to the sides; symptoms such as vertigo, diplopia, and nausea are positive signs.

Cervical spondylotic myelopathy

The main symptoms are:

- Sensory disturbance and dyskinesia. Symptoms characteristically start to manifest in the lower limbs as numbness, heaviness of one or both lower limbs, followed by difficulty walking and instability. Symptoms manifest next in the torso as sensory disturbance of the region below the ribs T2–4, and tightness in the region of the chest, abdomen, and pelvis. Finally, symptoms manifest in the upper limbs as numbness, pain, asthenia of one or both upper limbs. Patients are unable to perform fine movement, even unable to take food by themselves.

- Restricted mobility in bending the head backwards and to the sides, tender spots on spinous processes and the muscles on both sides.

- A likelihood of hypermyotonia, tendon hyperreflexia; positive sign of the patella and ankle clonus test; loss of decrease of superficial reflex, deep reflex exists; pathological indications such as positive sign of Hoffman's test (Figure 1.10), positive sign of Babinski's test (Figure 1.11).

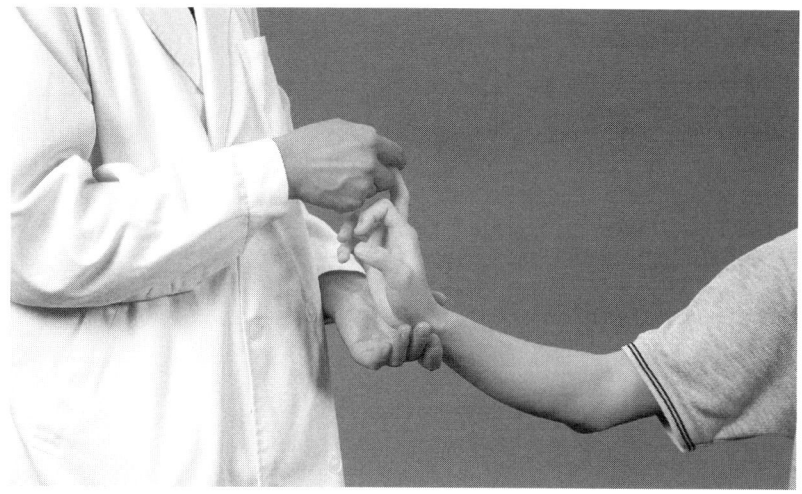

Figure 1.10 Hoffman's test

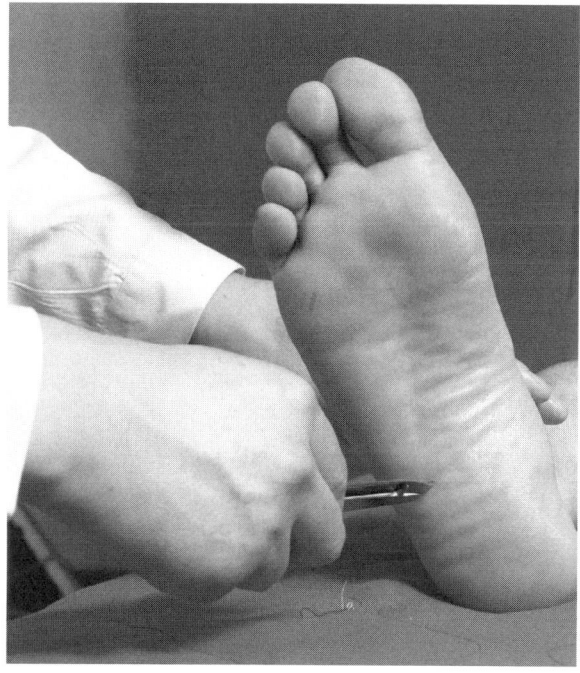

Figure 1.11 Babinski's test

Sympathetic cervical spondylosis

The main symptoms are:

- **Sympathetic excitation type of sympathetic cervical spondylosis:** Symptoms such as headache, vertigo, increase of oculi rimae (space between upper and lower eyelids), blurred vision, mydriasis, rapid heart rate, arrhythmia, precordial pain, raised blood pressure, vasospasm of limbs, partial hypothermia, hidrosis, tinnitus, slowed peristalsis of stomach and intestines.

- **Vagal excitation type of sympathetic cervical spondylosis:** Headache, vertigo, ptosis, ploration (excessive watering of the eye), snuffle, slow heart rate, reduced blood pressure, quickening of peristalsis of the stomach and intestines, or belching.

Chapter 2

Fundamentals of Treatment for Cervical Spondylosis

Section I Meridians and Collaterals

The system of meridians and collaterals connects the viscera, limbs, and orifices; it is the pathway for circulating qi and blood; it nourishes the whole body and protects it from exogenous harm. Pathogenic factors travel along the meridians and collaterals; they show manifestations of disease, reflect pathological changes, and the effects of direct treatment (Figure 2.1).

The path of meridians and collaterals related to cervical spondylosis is introduced below.

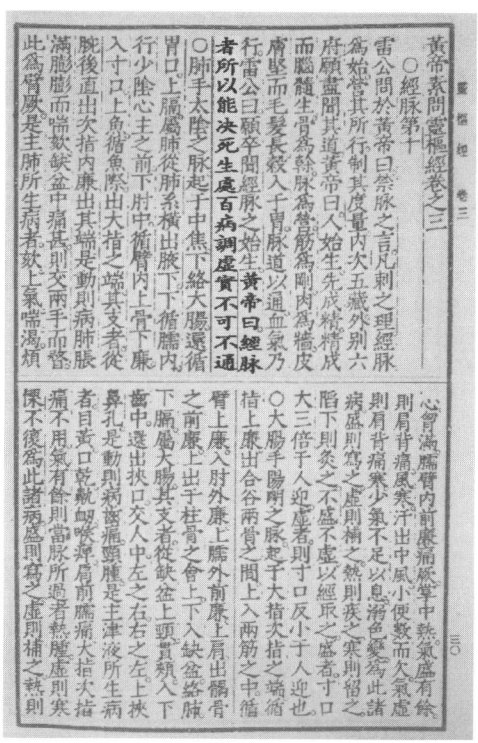

Figure 2.1 Recordation of ancient books

1. The Lung Meridian of Hand-Taiyin

From the lung system, which relates to the portion of the lung communicating with the throat, the meridian comes out transversely. Descending along the medial aspect of the upper arm, it passes in front of the Heart Meridian of Hand-Shaoyin and the Pericardium Meridian of Hand-Jueyin, and reaches the cubital fossa. Then it goes continuously downward along the anterior border of the radial side in the medial aspect of the forearm and enters *cunkou* (the radial artery at the wrist for pulse palpation). Passing the thenar eminence, it goes along its radial border, ending at the medial side of the tip of the thumb (Figure 2.2).

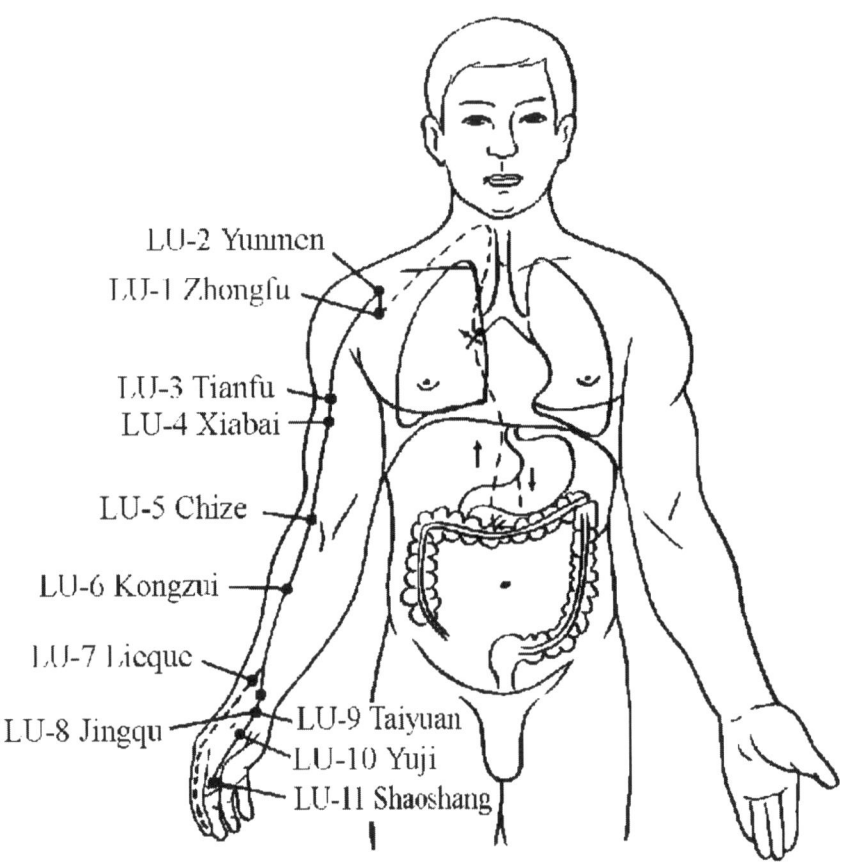

Figure 2.2 The Lung Meridian of Hand-Taiyin

2. The Large Intestine Meridian of Hand-Yangming

This meridian starts from the tip of the index finger. Running upward along the radial side of the index finger and passing through the space between the first and second metacarpal bones, it enters the depression between the tendons of m. extensor pollicis longus and brevis. Then, continuing along the anterior aspect of the forearm, it reaches the lateral side of the elbow. Then it ascends along the lateral anterior aspect of the upper arm to the highest point of the shoulder, along the anterior border of the acromion and up as far as the cervical vertebra, and descends to ST-12 Quepen (Figure 2.3).

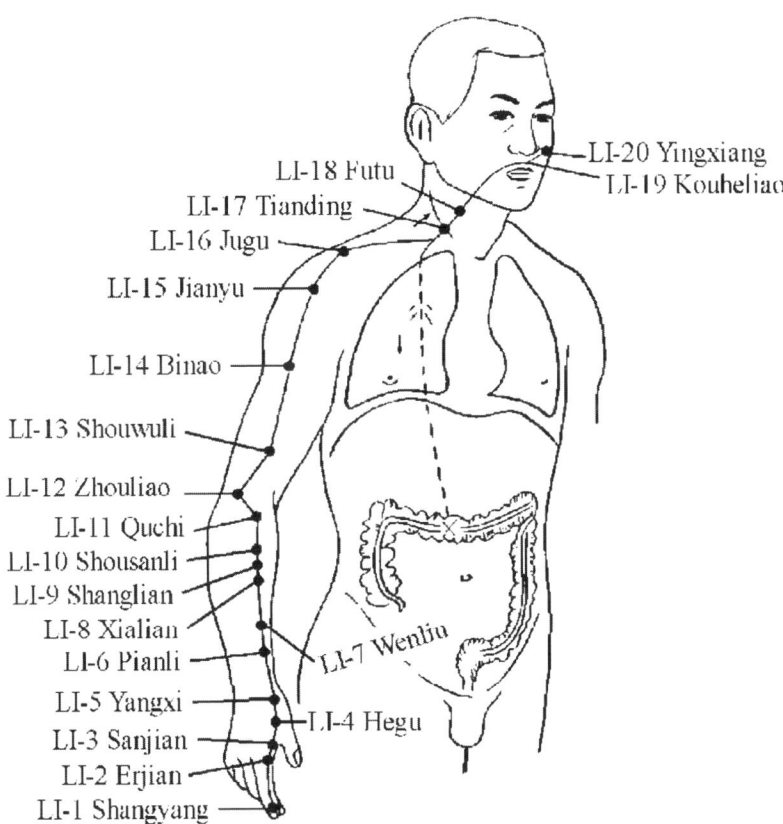

Figure 2.3 The Large Intestine Meridian of Hand-Yangming

3. The Heart Meridian of Hand-Shaoyin

The meridian runs out from the axilla and along the posterior border of the medial aspect of the upper arm, behind the Lung Meridian and Pericardium Meridian. It then runs down the medial aspect of the elbow and descends along the posterior border of the medial aspect of the forearm to the pisiform region proximal to the palm. Entering the palm, it follows the medial aspect of the little finger to its tip (Figure 2.4).

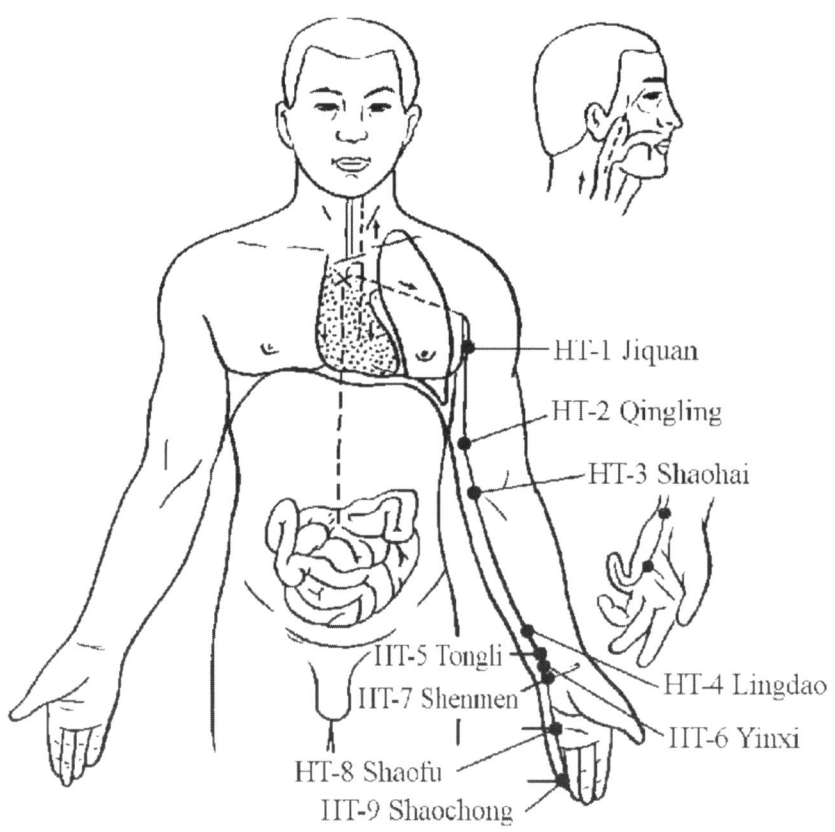

HT-1 Jiquan

HT-2 Qingling

HT-3 Shaohai

HT-4 Lingdao

HT-5 Tongli

HT-7 Shenmen

HT-6 Yinxi

HT-8 Shaofu

HT-9 Shaochong

Figure 2.4 The Heart Meridian of Hand-Shaoyin

4. The Small Intestine Meridian of Hand-Taiyang

The meridian starts from the ulnar side of the tip of the little finger. Following the ulnar side of the dorsum of the hand, it reaches the wrist. Then it goes out from the styloid process of the ulna, ascends along the posterior border of the lateral aspect of the forearm, passes between the olecranon of the ulna and the medial epicondyle of the humerus and runs along the posterior border of the lateral aspect of the upper arm to the shoulder joint. Circling around the scapular region, it meets the superior aspect of the shoulder, then turns downward to ST-12 Quepen (Figure 2.5).

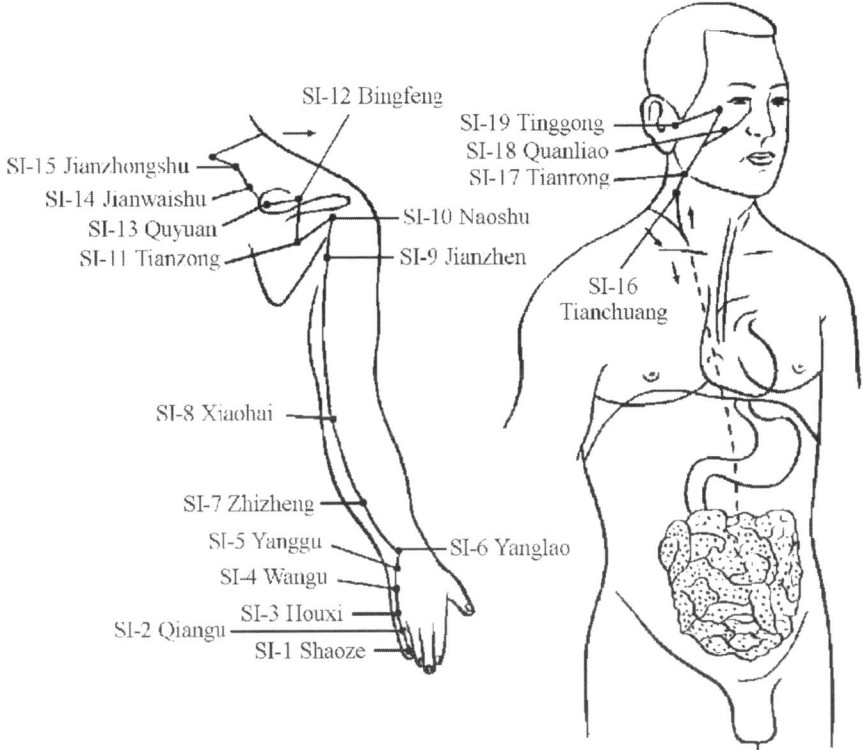

Figure 2.5 The Small Intestine Meridian of Hand-Taiyang

5. The Bladder Meridian of Foot-Taiyang

The meridian enters and communicates with the brain from the vertex, then comes out and bifurcates to descend along the posterior aspect of the neck, and down along the medial aspect of the scapula region, parallel to the vertebral column. It reaches the lumbar region (Figure 2.6).

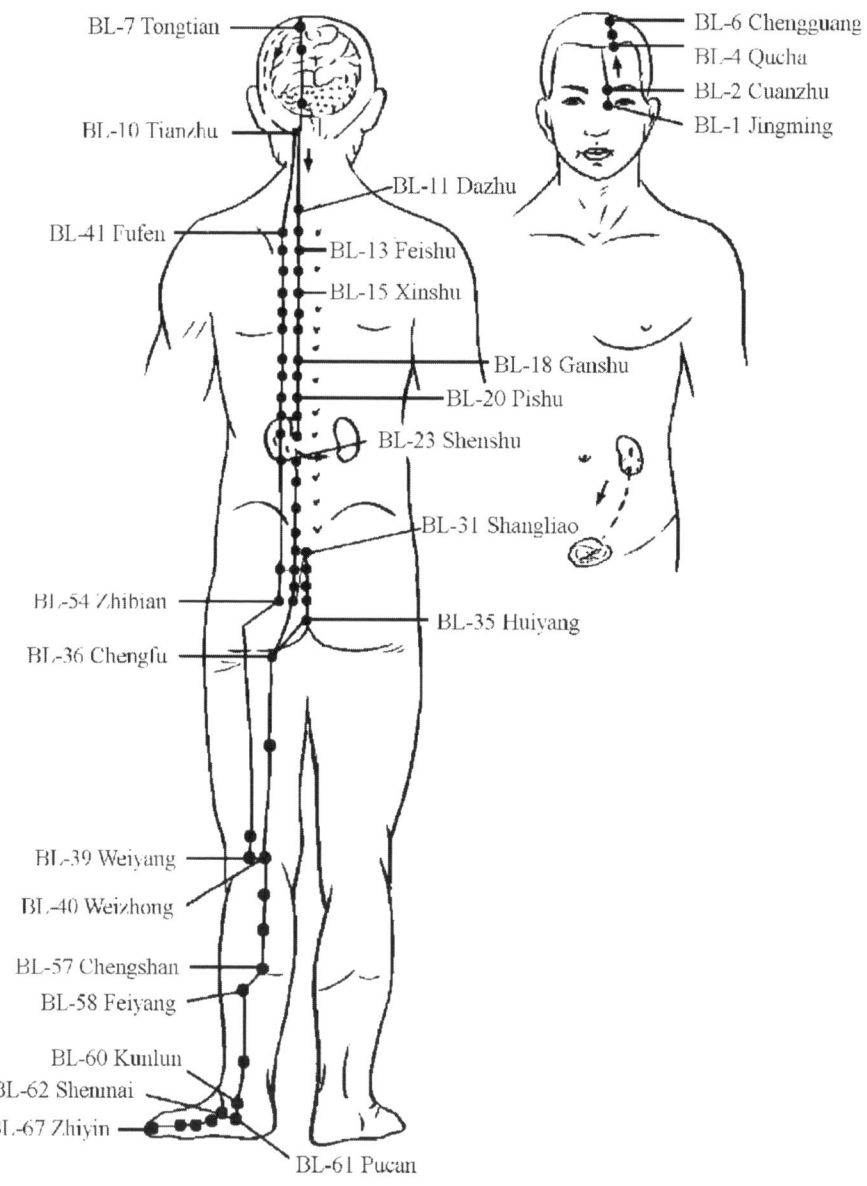

Figure 2.6 The Bladder Meridian of Foot-Taiyang

6. The Pericardium Meridian of Hand-Jueyin

The meridian begins below the axilla and ascends to the axilla. Following the medial aspect of the upper arm, it runs between the Lung Meridian and Heart Meridian to the cubital fossa, down to the forearm between the tendons of m. palmaris longus and m. flexor carpi radialis, enters the palm, then passes along the middle finger right down to its tip (Figure 2.7).

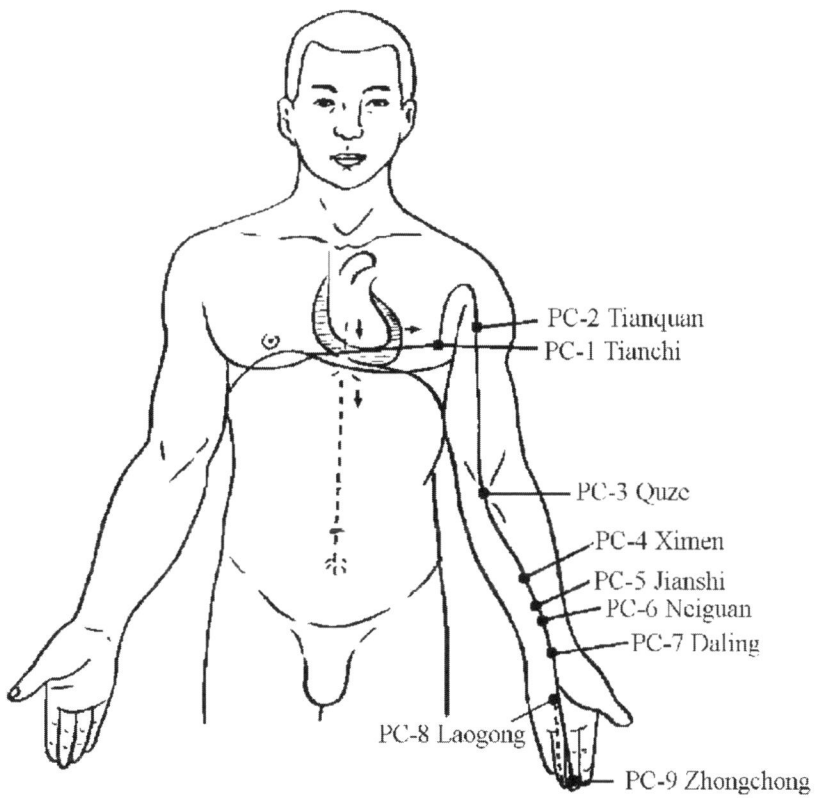

Figure 2.7 The Pericardium Meridian of Hand-Jueyin

7. The Sanjiao Meridian of Hand-Shaoyang

Originating from the tip of the ring finger, the meridian runs upward between the fourth and fifth metacarpal bones, along the dorsal aspect of the wrist to the lateral aspect of the forearm between the radius and ulna, then ascends through the olecranon and goes along the lateral aspect of the upper arm, reaches the shoulder region, crosses it, and passes behind the Gallbladder Meridian, winding over to ST-12 Quepen (Figure 2.8).

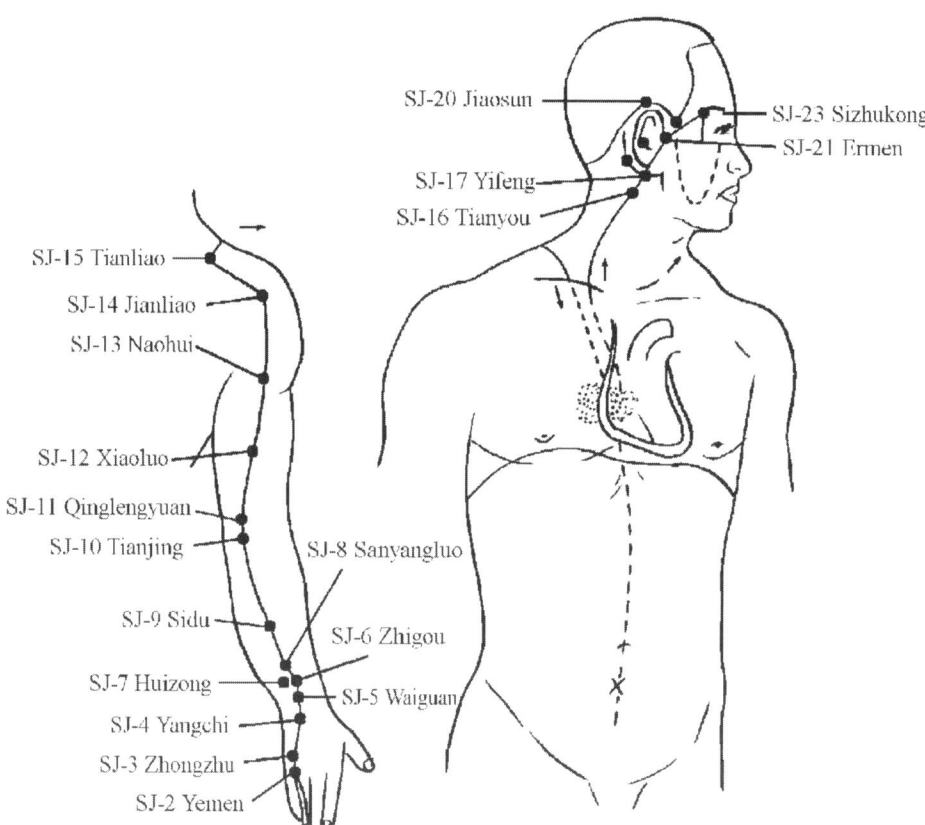

Figure 2.8 The Sanjiao Meridian of Hand-Shaoyang

8. The Gallbladder Meridian of Foot-Shaoyang

The meridian ascends to the corner of the forehead, then curves downward to the retroauricular region and round along the side of the neck in front of the Triple Burner Meridian to the shoulder. It then turns back, traverses and passes behind the Triple Burner Meridian, down to the ST-12 Quepen (Figure 2.9).

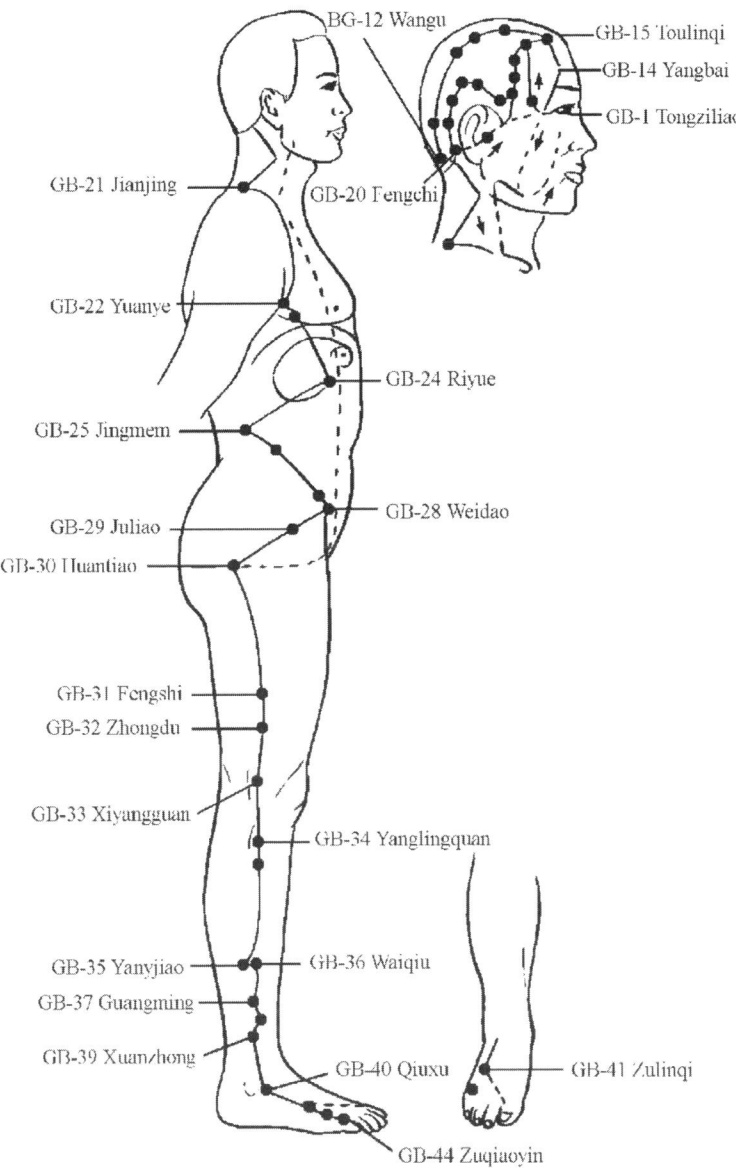

Figure 2.9 The Gallbladder Meridian of Foot-Shaoyang

9. Governor Vessel

Governor Vessel arises from the lower abdomen and comes out from the perineum. It runs posteriorly along the interior side of the spinal column to DU-16 Fengfu at the nape, where it enters the brain. It further ascends to the vertex and then goes down along the forehead to the nasal column (Figure 2.10).

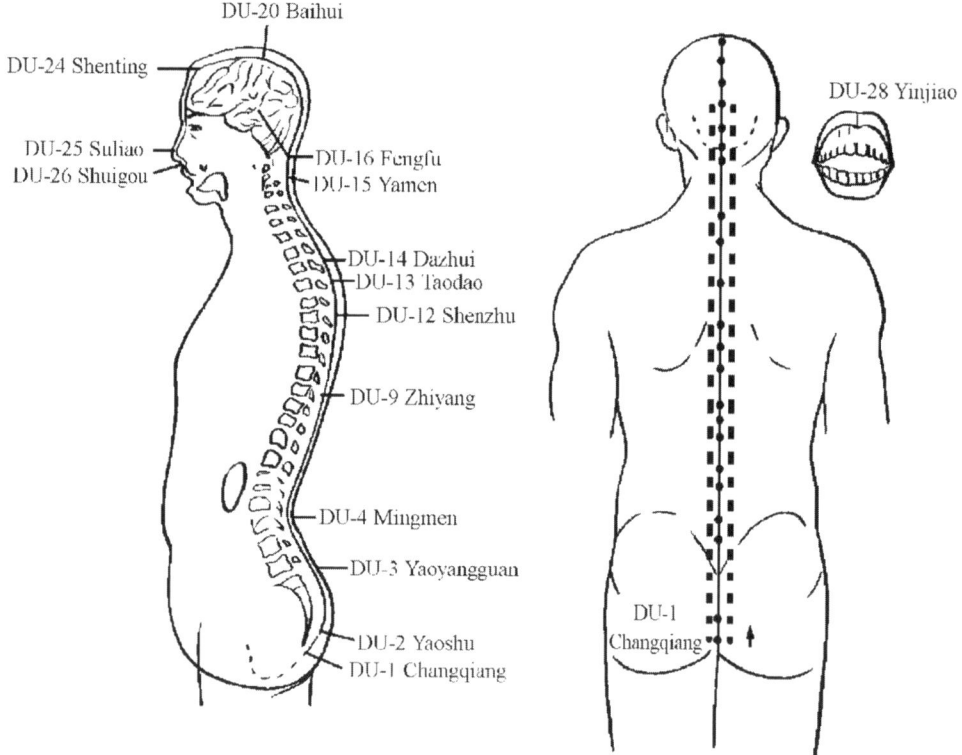

Figure 2.10 The Governor Vessel

Section II Acupoints

1. The Large Intestine Meridian of Hand-Yangming

The acupoints of the Large Intestine Meridian of Hand-Yangming are shown in Figure 2.11.

- **LI-4 Hegu:** On the dorsum of the hand, between the first and second metacarpal bones, and on the radial side of the midpoint of the second metacarpal bone.

- **LI-10 Shousanli:** On the radial side of the dorsal surface of the forearm and 2 cun below the cubital crease, on the line connecting LI-5 Yangxi and LI-11 Quchi.

- **LI-11 Quchi:** With the elbow flexed, at the lateral end of the cubital crease, at the midpoint of the line connecting LU-5 Chize and external humeral epicondyle.

- **LI-14 Binao:** On the lateral side of the arm, at the insertion of deltoid muscle and on the line connecting LI-11 Quchi and LI-15 Jianyu, 7 cun above LI-11 Quchi.

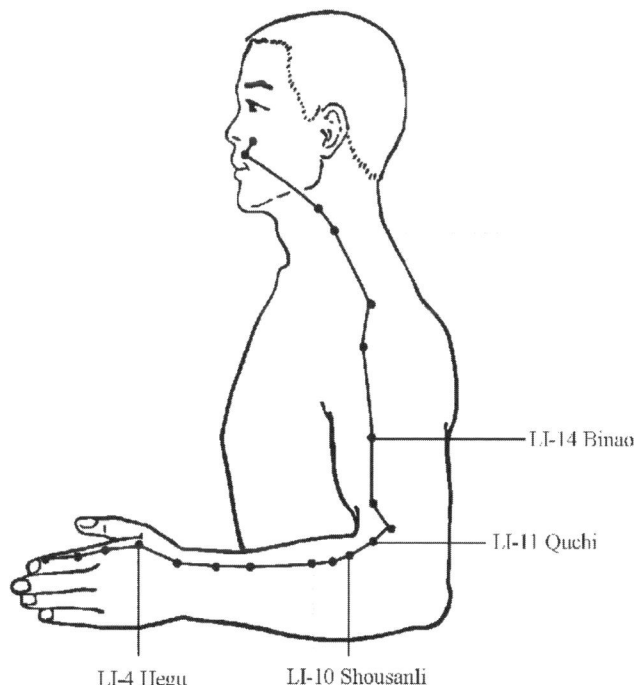

Figure 2.11 Acupoints of the Large Intestine Meridian of Hand-Yangming

2. The Stomach Meridian of Foot-Yangming

The acupoints of the Stomach Meridian of Foot-Yangming are shown in Figure 2.12.

- **ST-8 Touwei:** On the head, 0.5 cun above the anterior hairline at the corner of the forehead, and 4.5 cun lateral to the midline of the head.

- **ST-12 Quepen:** In the lateral external region of the nape, at the centre of the supraclavicular fossa (the depression on the superior edge of the clavicle), 4 cun lateral to the anterior midline.

- **ST-36 Zusanli:** On the anterior lateral side of the leg, 3 cun below ST-35 Dubi, one finger breadth (middle finger) from the anterior crest of the tibia.

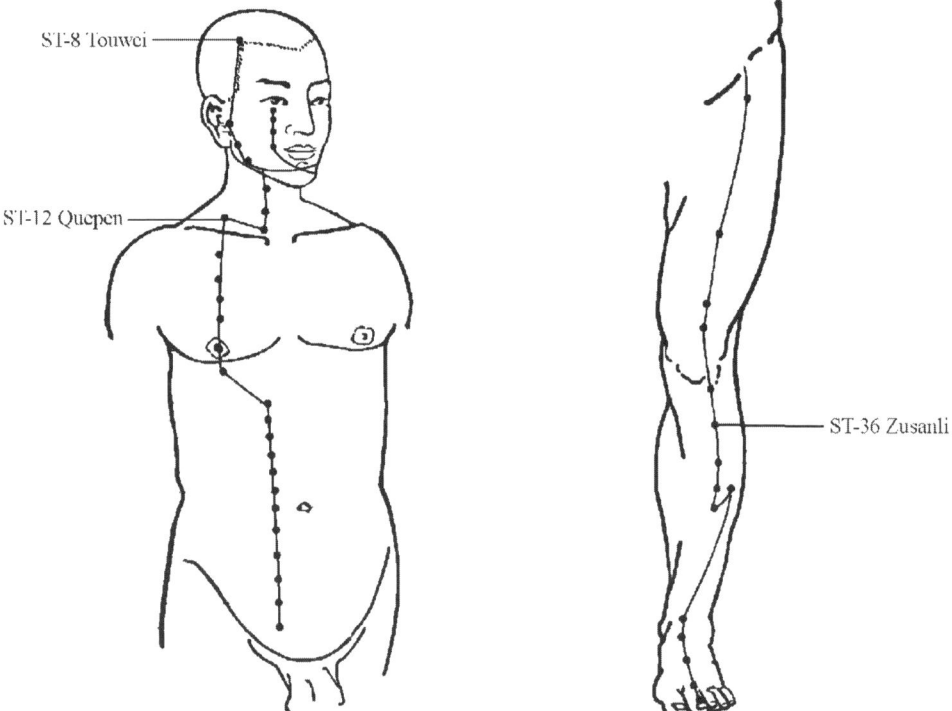

Figure 2.12 Acupoints of the Stomach Meridian of Foot-Yangming

3. The Spleen Meridian of Foot-Taiyin

The acupoints of the Spleen Meridian of Foot-Taiyin are shown in Figure 2.13.

• **SP-6 Sanyinjiao:** On the medial side of the leg, 3 cun above the tip of the medial malleolus, posterior to the medial border of the tibia.

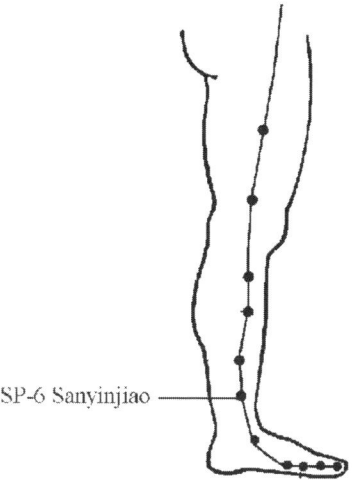

*Figure 2.13 Acupoints of the Spleen
Meridian of Foot-Taiyin*

4. The Heart Meridian of Hand-Shaoyin

The acupoints of the Heart Meridian of Hand-Shaoyin are shown in Figure 2.14.

• **HT-1 Jiquan:** At the centre of the axillary fossa, where the pulsation of the axillary artery is palpable.

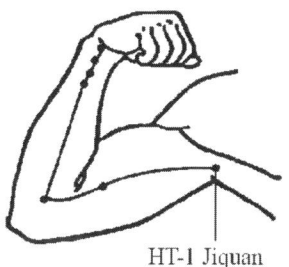

*Figure 2.14 Acupoints of the Heart
Meridian of Hand-Shaoyin*

5. The Small Intestine Meridian of Hand-Taiyang

The acupoints of the Small Intestine Meridian of Hand-Taiyang are shown in Figure 2.15.

- **SI-3 Houxi:** At the junction of the red and white skin along the ulnar border of the hand, at the ulnar end of the distal palmar crease, proximal to the fifth metacarpophalangeal joint when a hollow fist is made.

- **SI-8 Xiaohai:** On the medial side of the elbow, in the depression between the olecranon of the ulna and the medial epicondyle of the humerus.

- **SI-9 Jianzhen:** On the scapula, posterior and inferior to the shoulder joint, 1 cun above the posterior end of the axillary fold with the arm adducted.

- **SI-11 Tianzong:** On the scapula, in the depression of the centre of the subscapular fossa, level with the fourth thoracic vertebra.

- **SI-15 Jianzhongshu:** On the back, below the spinous process of the seventh cervical vertebra, 2 cun lateral to the posterior midline.

- **SI-14 Jianwaishu:** On the spine, below the spinous process of the first thoracic vertebra, 3 cun lateral to the posterior midline.

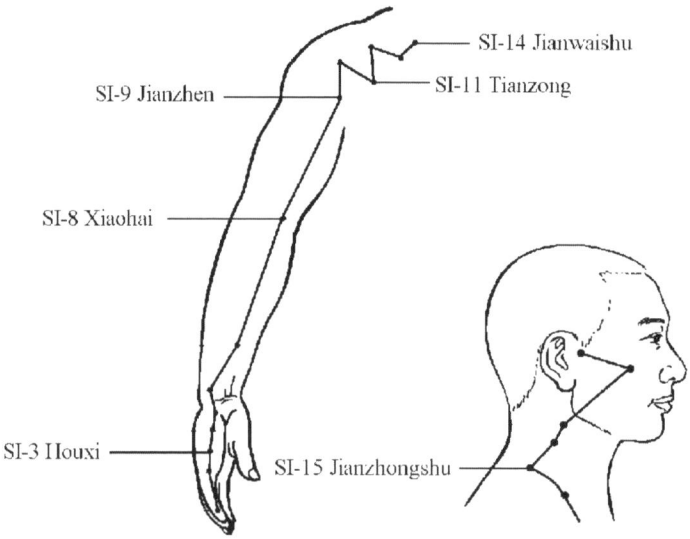

Figure 2.15 Acupoints of the Small Intestine Meridian of Hand-Taiyang

6. The Bladder Meridian of Foot-Taiyang

The acupoints of the Bladder Meridian of Foot-Taiyang are shown in Figure 2.16.

- **BL-39 Weiyang:** On the knee, on the popliteal crease, medial to the tendon of the biceps muscle of the thigh.

- **BL-40 Weizhong:** At the midpoint of the popliteal crease, between the tendon of the biceps muscle of the thigh and the semitendinosus muscle.

- **BL-54 Zhibian:** On the sacrum, on the level of the fourth posterior sacral foramen, 3 cun lateral to the median sacral crest.

- **BL-57 Chengshan:** On the posterior midline of the calf, between BL-40 Weizhong and BL-60 Kunlun, a pointed depression formed below the belly of the gastrocnemius muscle when the leg is stretched or the heel is lifted.

- **BL-60 Kunlun:** Posterior to the lateral malleolus, in the depression between the tip of the external malleolus and the Achilles tendon.

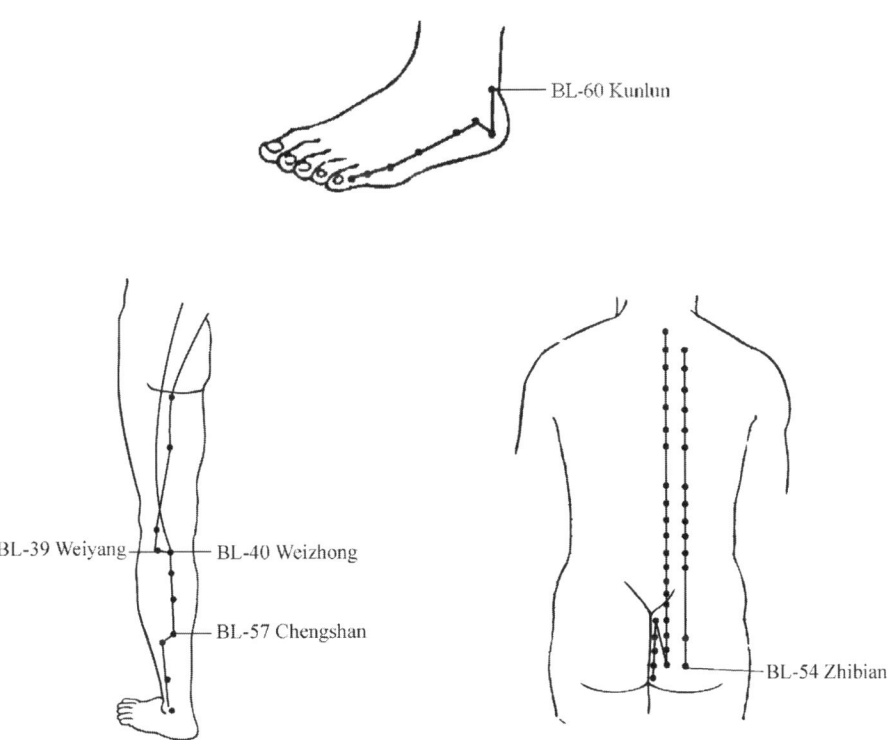

Figure 2.16 Acupoints of the Bladder Meridian of Foot-Taiyang

7. The Kidney Meridian of Foot-Shaoyin

The acupoints of the Kidney Meridian of Foot-Shaoyin are shown in Figure 2.17.

- **KI-1 Yongquan:** On the thenar, in the depression appearing on the anterior part of the sole when the foot is in plantar flexion.

- **KI-3 Taixi:** Posterior to the medial malleolus, in the depression between the tip of the medial malleolus and Achilles tendon.

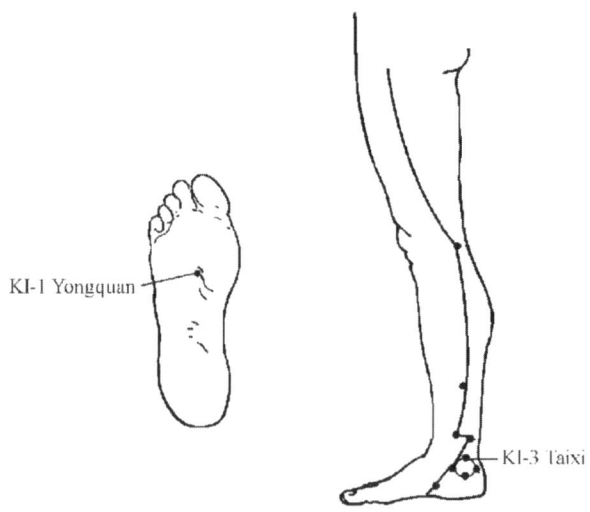

Figure 2.17 Acupoints of the Kidney Meridian of Foot-Shaoyin

8. The Pericardium Meridian of Hand-Jueyin

The acupoints of the Pericardium Meridian of Hand-Jueyin are shown in Figure 2.18.

- **PC-6 Neiguan:** On the palmar side of the forearm, 2 cun above the crease of the wrist, between the tendon of palmaris longus and the tendon of flexor carpi radialis.

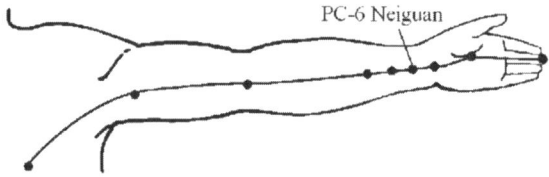

Figure 2.18 Acupoints of the Pericardium Meridian of Hand-Jueyin

9. The Sanjiao Meridian of Hand-Shaoyang

The acupoints of the Sanjiao Meridian of Hand-Shaoyanng are shown in Figure 2.19.

- **TE-5 Waiguan:** On the dorsal side of the forearm, 2 cun proximal to the dorsal crease of the wrist, at the centre of the space between the radius and ulna.

- **TE-20 Jiaosun:** On the head, above the ear apex, within the hairline.

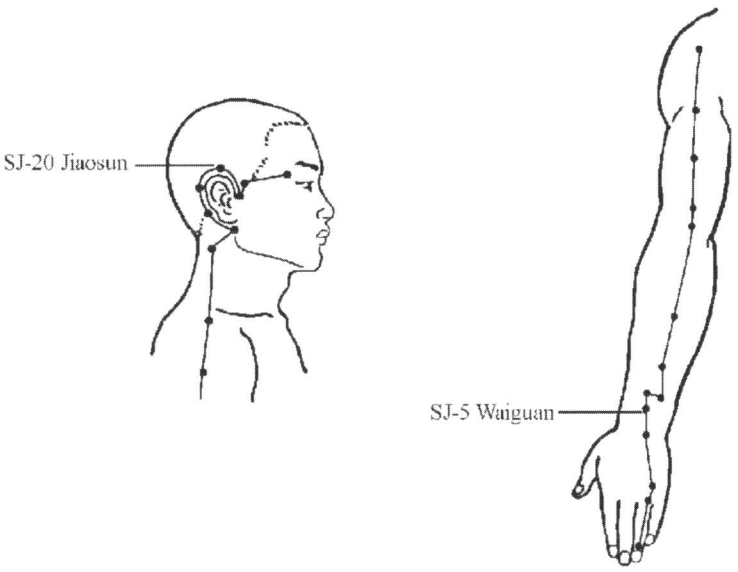

Figure 2.19 Acupoints of the Sanjiao Meridian of Hand-Shaoyang

10. The Gallbladder Meridian of Foot-Shaoyang

The acupoints of the Gallbladder Meridian of Foot Shaoyang are shown in Figure 2.20.

- **GB-21 Jianjing:** On the scapula, at the midpoint of the line connecting the spinous process of C7 and the lateral point of the acromion.

- **GB-30 Huantiao:** On the buttock, at the junction of the middle third and lateral third of the line between the prominence of the great trochanter and the sacral hiatus, when the patient is in a lateral recumbent position with the thigh flexed.

- **GB-34 Yanglingquan:** On the lateral side of the shank, in a depression anterior and inferior to the head of the fibula.

- **GB-39 Xuanzhong:** On the lateral side of shank, 3 cun above the tip of the external malleolus, on the anterior border of the fibula.

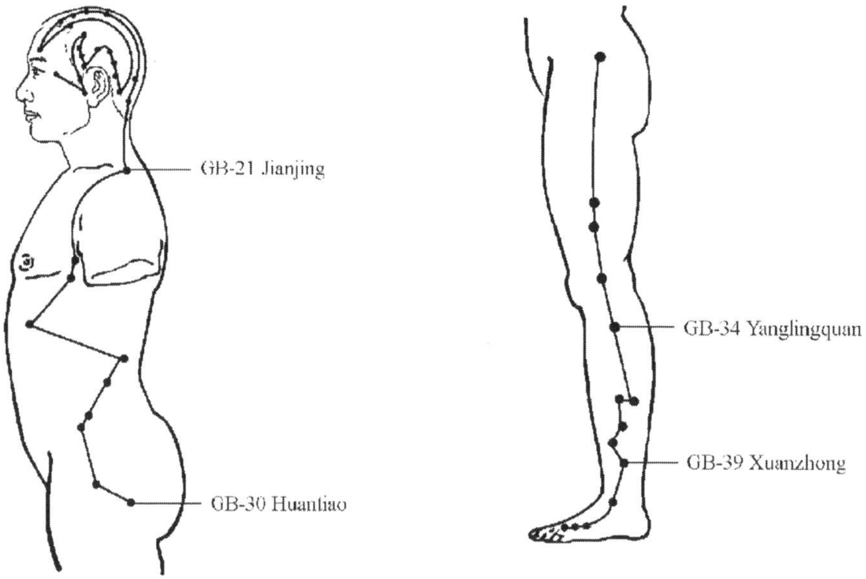

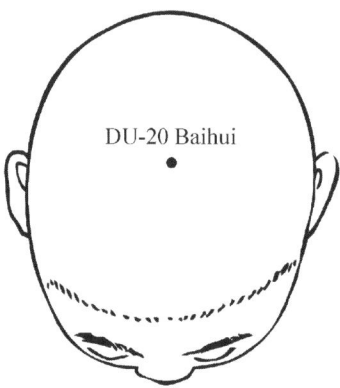

Figure 2.20 Acupoints of the Gallbladder Meridian of Foot-Shaoyang

11. The Governor Vessel

The acupoints of the Governor Vessel are shown in Figure 2.21.

- **DU-20 Baihui:** On the head, 5 cun directly above the midpoint of the anterior hairline.

Figure 2.21 Acupoints of the Governor Vessel

12. The Conception Vessel

The acupoints of the Conception Vessel are shown in Figure 2.22.

- **RN-12 Zhongwan:** On the anterior midline, 4 cun above the centre of the umbilicus.

- **RN-17 Danzhong:** On the anterior midline, level with the fourth intercostal space, at the midpoint of the line joining the nipples.

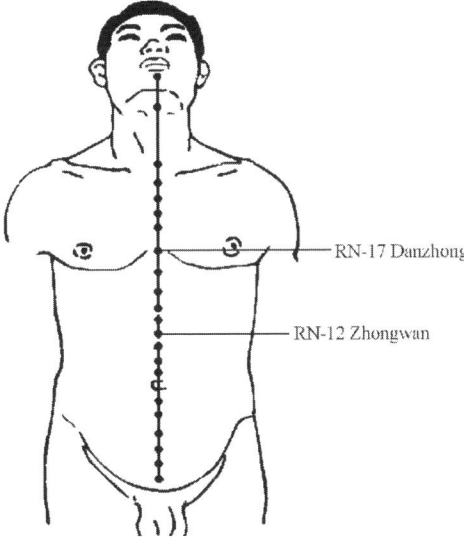

Figure 2.22 Acupoints of the Conception Vessel

13. The Extraordinary points

The Extraordinary points are shown in Figure 2.23.

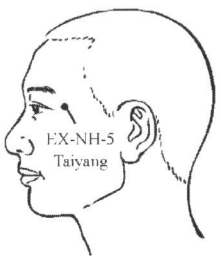

- **EX-HN-5 Taiyang:** On the head, between the lateral end of the eyebrow and the outer canthus, in the depression one finger breadth behind them.

- **EX-HN-1 Sishencong:** On the top of the head, 1 cun anterior, posterior and lateral to DU-20 Baihui (four acupoints altogether).

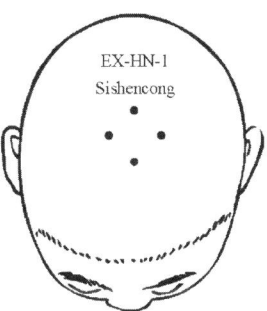

Figure 2.23 The Extraordinary points

Section III Anatomy

The intervertebral foramen

The intervertebral foramen (Figure 2.24) is a diagonal, bony aperture that allows for the passage of the spinal nerve root. The intervertebral foramen can be examined by means of an oblique X-ray view of the cervical spine, because it is diagonal. The longitudinal diameter of the intervertebral foramen is greater than its transverse diameter, and the volume of the nerve root is half that of the space provided by the intervertebral foramen. When there is a degeneration of the cervical spine and narrowing of the intervertebral space, the nerve root will not initially be compressed; but when there is degeneration of the cervical spine with horizontal subluxation, then the nerve root is liable to be stimulated.

The medial wall of the intervertebral foramen is the uncovertebral joint, and its lateral wall is the intervertebral joint of the cervical spine. The superior and inferior walls are formed by notches in the pedicle of the vertebral arc, thus creating the bony aperture known as the intervertebral foramen. When there is a displacement or hyperplasia of the medial wall (uncovertebral joint) and lateral wall (intervertebral joint) of the intervertebral foramen, the nerve root within the intervertebral foramen will be stimulated.

As there are no intervertebral discs between the occipital bone and C1, or between C1 and C2, there are no intervertebral foramina to protect the first and second nerve roots, so they are particularly vulnerable.

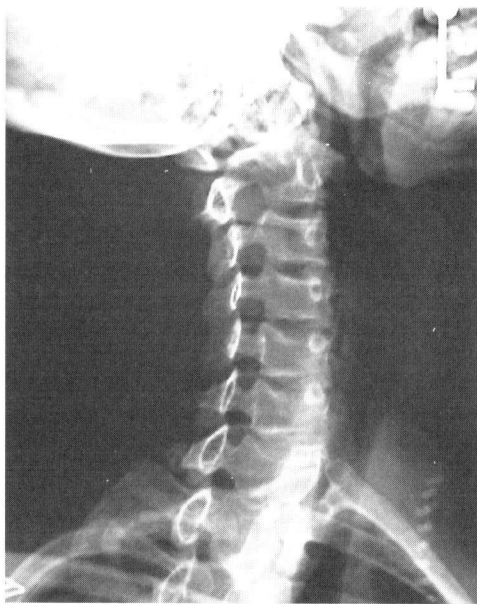

Figure 2.24 Intervertebral foramen

The vertebral artery

The vertebral artery (Figure 2.25) is the first branch of the subclavian artery. Sometimes it originates from the aortic arch or innominate artery. There is asymmetry between the vertebral arteries on either side: normally the left one is bigger, and the right one smaller. The vertebral artery can be divided into four parts, as described below.

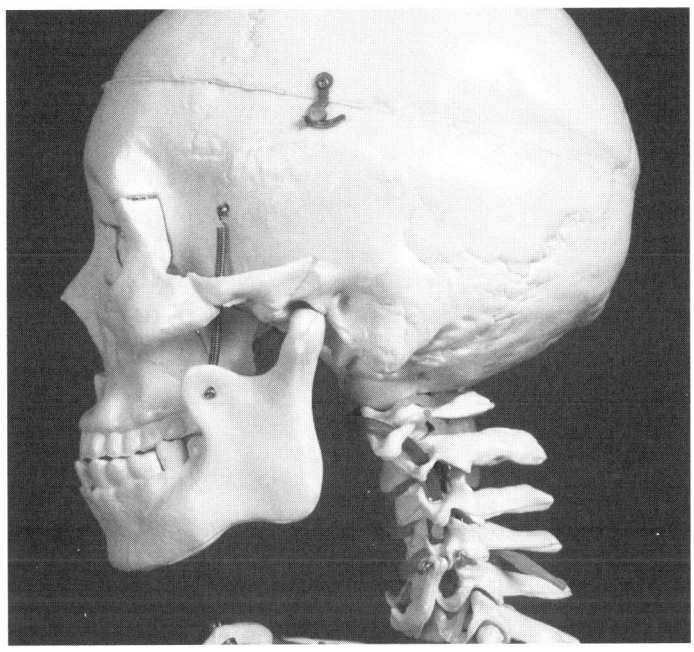

Figure 2.25 Vertebral artery

1. FIRST PART (CERVICAL PART)

The first part originates from the subclavian artery, and runs upward in the cranny between the longus colli and the scalenus anterior. Behind it, it is crossed by the vertebral vein, jugular vein, common carotid artery, and superior thyroid artery. Behind it there are also the seventh and eighth ventral ramus of the cervical nerve and the transverse process of the seventh cervical vertebra, which lies next to the sympathetic trunk and the inferior cervical ganglion. Sympathetic fibers originating from the inferior cervical ganglion lie alongside the vertebral artery, so, clinically, compression of the vertebral artery can be caused by spasm of scalenus anterior, and symptoms of both cervical spondylotic radiculopathy and of the vertebral artery type of cervical spondylosis can be seen simultaneously.

2. SECOND PART (SPINAL CANAL PART)

The second part runs upward through the foramina in the transverse processes of the upper six cervical vertebrae. The cervical artery in this part is in front of the second to sixth ventral ramus of the cervical nerve, and is surrounded by a plexus of nerves and veins. On the medial side of the cervical artery are uncovertebral joints. The cervical artery is liable to be stimulated, stretched, compressed, or distorted when there is hyperplasia of the uncovertebral joints or displacement of vertebrae, leading to stenosis of the cervical artery, and restricted flow of blood. The artery may even become obstructed causing cataplexy, if hyperplasia or displacement is severe.

3. THIRD PART (INFERIOR CEPHALIC PART)

Issues from the transverse foramen of the atlas, and curves backward behind the lateral mass of the atlas; it then lies in the groove on the upper surface of the posterior arch of the atlas, and enters the vertebral canal by passing beneath the external border of the posterior atlanto-occipital membrane. It then goes upward, and into the skull through the foramen magnum. The vertebral artery is very sinuous at this part, so it is liable to be stretched by rotation of head, and this may lead to the symptoms of ischemia.

4. FOURTH PART (ENCEPHALIC PART)

Goes upward along the medial side of the medulla oblongata, through foramen magnum. At the lower border of the pons the vertebral artery from one side unites with the one from the opposite side to form the basilar artery. The encephalic branches of the blood vessel are the terminal portion of the vertebral artery, the anterior spinal artery, posterior inferior cerebellar artery, posterior spinal artery, and the artery of inner ear. The artery of inner ear (labyrinthine artery) is a long, slender, circuitous branch of the vertebrobasilar artery, and is distributed to the internal ear, so when there is a vertebral artery type of cervical spondylosis, there will be a vertebrobasilar artery insufficiency, and the patient's clinical manifestations are tinnitus, dysacousis, etc.

The brachial plexus

The brachial plexus (Figure 2.26) is formed by the anterior branch of the spinal nerves of C5–C8 and part of the anterior branch of the spinal nerve of T1, and it supplies the muscles and skin of the upper arm. It passes between the anterior and middle scalene muscles, continues above the subclavian artery, past the clavicle, and enters the axilla. In the axilla, it follows the axillary artery and forms the medial cord, lateral cord, and posterior cord. The brachial plexus is separated by the clavicle, into the supraclavicular division and the infraclavicular division.

It concentrates on the upper part of the midpoint of clavical and axillary, where anesthesia can be injected.

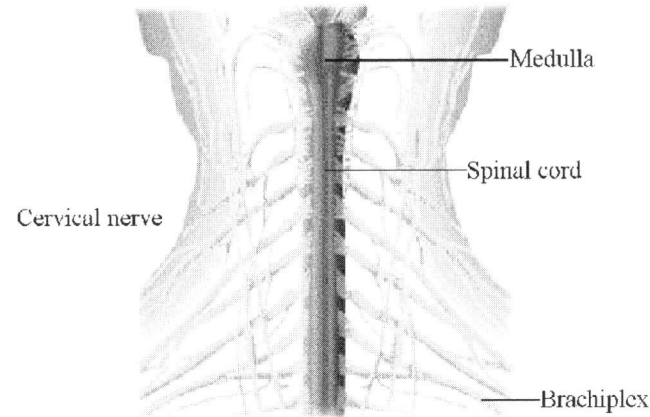

Figure 2.26 Cervical spinal nerves

The cervical spinal cord

The spinal cord is located in the vertebral canal. It is ovoid-shaped. Its upper part is enlarged and connects with the medulla in the region of the foramen magnum. The lower part is smaller and becomes cone-shaped, so it is called the terminal cone.

A long, thin filament, called the terminal filament, extends from the terminal part of the cone.

The cervical spinal cord connects with the medulla. Both its inner structure and its physiological functionality can hardly be differentiated from those of the lower medulla. Coma can occur when there is injury of the upper cervical spinal cord.

The longitudinal diameter of the cervical spinal cord is less than its transverse diameter. It is enlarged in the region of C2–T2, especially C5–C6, because this part of the spinal cord supplies the upper limbs and hands, and its functionality here is multiple and complex.

Section IV Manipulations

Pushing manipulation with one finger

METHOD

Exert force through the entire surface of the thumb to act on one side of the neck; the four fingers are placed on the other side of the neck. Flex and extend the interphalangeal joint and sway the wrist, so as to make the force act on the area to be treated (Figure 2.27).

THE MOVEMENT

- Drop the shoulder: relax the shoulder and let it drop, no lifting up, no abduction.

- Drop the elbow: the elbow drops naturally.

- Fixation of finger: the part on which the force is exerted should be fixed on the spot to be treated.

- Push forcefully and move slowly: forceful pushing means that the frequency of swaying is fairly high, normally 140 times per minute; moving slowly means that the movements to-and-fro between one treated point and the other should be slow.

- Generate force with the palm, transmit force with the thumb, exerting force on the entire surface of the thumb: the force of this technique is generated by the palm, transmitted by the thumb through its entire surface, and acts on the surface of the patient's body. By exerting the force in this way, it is contained within and not manifested outside.

FUNCTION

This technique affects the muscle layer, and has the function of releasing muscle spasm.

NOTE

During this procedure, flexion and extension of the thumb and swaying of the wrist should be in unison.

This technique may be done both forcefully and softly, but mainly forcefully. During the treatment, the treated points form a line, and lines form a surface, so that the whole treated area can be relaxed.

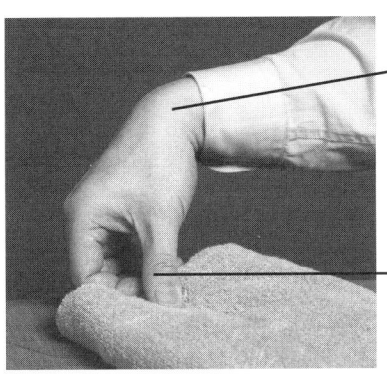

Wrist swings laterally

Extension of interphalangeal joint

Swing laterally

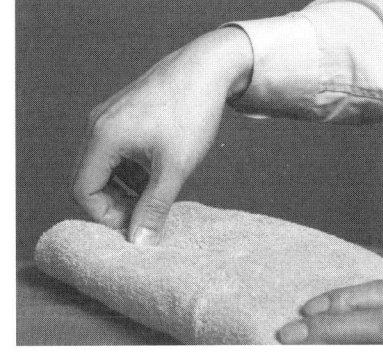

Neutral position

Wrist swings medially

Flexion of interphalangeal joints

Swing medially

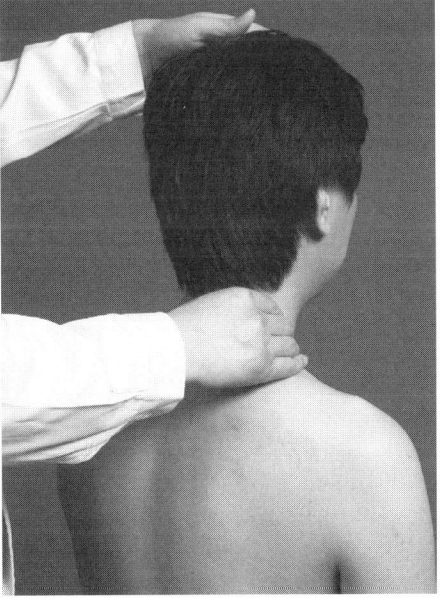

Figure 2.27 Pushing manipulation with one finger

Rolling manipulation

METHOD

- **Lateral rolling:** The dorsal aspect of the hand, close to the little finger, rests on the spot to be treated. The dorsal aspect of the metacarpophalangeal joint of the little finger is the pivot. Bend the elbow slightly and relax: rotating the forearm and flexing and extending the wrist joint, exert force to continuously act on the spot to be treated (Figure 2.28).

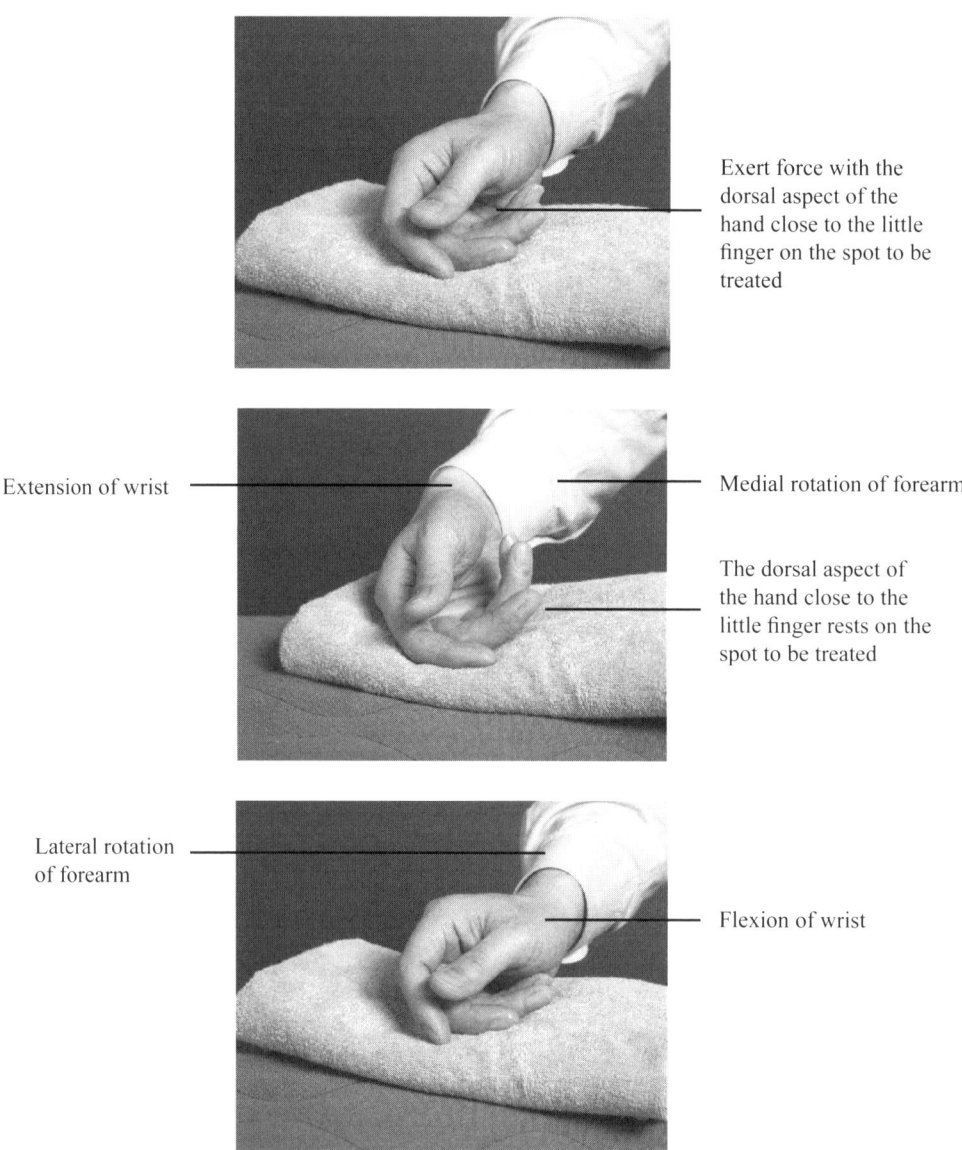

Exert force with the dorsal aspect of the hand close to the little finger on the spot to be treated

Extension of wrist

Medial rotation of forearm

The dorsal aspect of the hand close to the little finger rests on the spot to be treated

Lateral rotation of forearm

Flexion of wrist

Figure 2.28 Lateral rolling

- **Vertical rolling:** The dorsal aspect of the little finger, ring finger, and middle finger, and the metacarpophalangeal joints of these fingers rest on the spot to be treated. The dorsal aspect of the metacarpophalangeal joint of the little finger is the pivot. Extend the elbow, and by rotating the forearm and flexing and extending the wrist joint, exert the force to act continuously on the treated spot (Figure 2.29).

THE MOVEMENT

- The part of the hand through which the force is exerted is likely to be spherical or bottle-shaped.

- The part of the hand on which the force is exerted rests on the area to be treated, with no forward or backward dragging.

- The elbow is slightly bent and the upper arm relaxed while doing *lateral* rolling; the elbow is extended while doing *vertical* rolling.

- The range of rolling is about 120° in *lateral* rolling; that is to say, roll laterally at an angle of 80° with the wrist bent; roll medially at an angle of 40° with the wrist extended. The range of rolling is about 45° when doing *vertical* rolling; that is to say, roll between the neutral position of the wrist and the dorsiflexed position with the wrist at an angle of 45°.

- Rotation of the forearm and flexion and extension of the wrist should be in unison when doing lateral rolling; that is to say, rotate the forearm outwards, bend the wrist joint, roll laterally; rotate the forearm inwards, dorsiflex the wrist joint, roll medially.

FUNCTION

This technique affects the muscle layer, and has the function of releasing muscle spasm.

NOTE

During the procedure, flexion and extension of the wrist and rotation of the forearm should be in unison.

This technique may be done both forcefully and softly, but mainly softly. The interface between the hand and the area to be treated is large, the pressure is high. Passive movement of the nape can be integrated when this technique is applied to the nape, so as to expand the range of movement of the joints during the process of relaxation, without causing pain in the process.

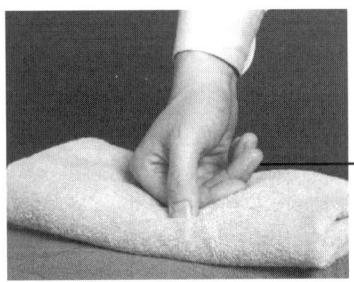

Exert force with the dorsal aspect of the little finger, ring finger, middle finger, and metacarpophalangeal joints of these fingers on the spot to be treated

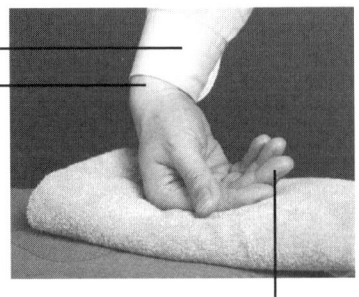

Lateral rotation of forearm

Flexion of wrist

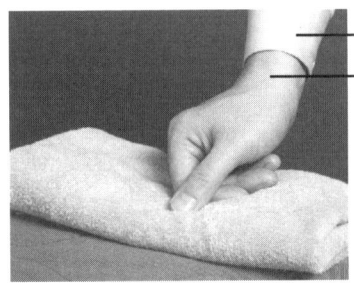

Medial rotation of forearm

Extension of wrist

The dorsal aspect of the little finger, ring finger, middle finger and metacapophalangeal joints of these fingers rest on the spot to be treated

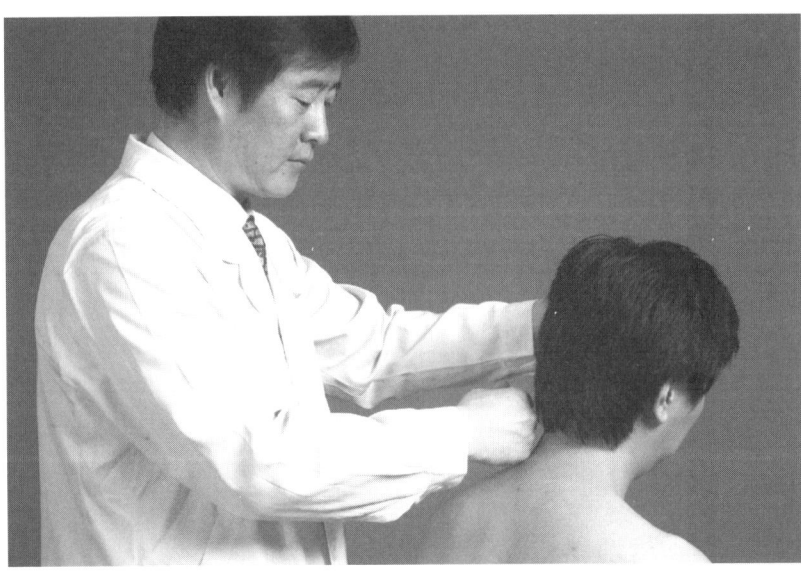

Figure 2.29 Vertical rolling

Kneading manipulation

METHOD

- **Finger kneading:** Rest the tips of the fingers on the area to be treated, and make gentle circular movements (Figure 2.30).

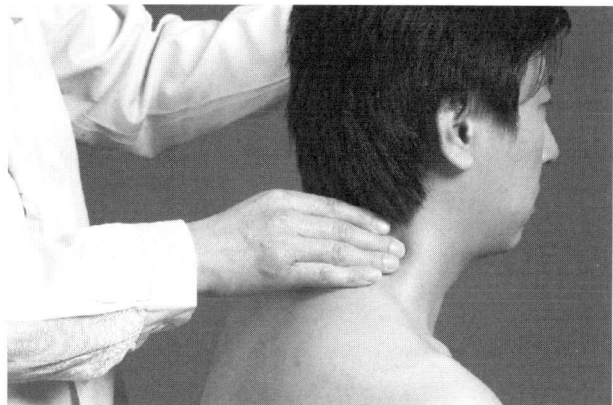

Figure 2.30 Kneading with the fingers

- **Palm kneading:** Exert force on the area to be treated with the palm, in gentle circular movements (Figure 2.31).

Rotating movement with fingers resting on the spot to be treated

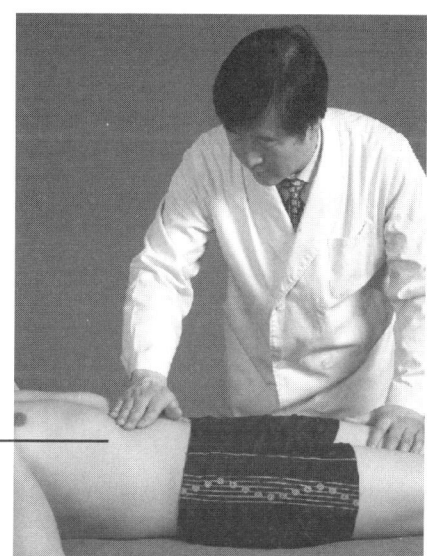

Figure 2.31 Kneading with the palms of the hands

THE MOVEMENT

- Move the proximal part of limb initially and then the distal part of limb to do the small, circular kneading. For example, move the forearm initially and then use the wrist, palm, and fingers to do the kneading.

- The part on which the force is exerted should rest on the spot to be treated, and should cause deeper layers of tissue to move.

- The pressure should be even; movement should be harmonious and rhythmic.

- The range of kneading should be moderate; either too large or too small a range is inadvisable.

FUNCTION

This technique acts on the muscle layer, and has the function of releasing muscle spasm and easing pain in the injured part.

NOTE

The part of the hand on which the force is exerted should be in contact with the spot to be treated. The range of kneading should be moderate. If the range is either too large or too small, it will impair relaxation.

This technique is gentle, slow, and soft; the stimulus is moderate, and can be applied to any part of the body.

Rubbing the abdomen

METHOD

Place the palm on the abdomen, and make circular, rhythmic rubbing movements. The normal sequence is: stomach – upper abdomen – navel – lower abdomen – lower right abdomen – upper right abdomen – upper left abdomen – lower left abdomen (Figure 2.32).

THE MOVEMENT

- Relax the upper limb, wrist, and palm, and place the hand lightly on the spot to be treated.

- Move the forearm initially and then use wrist and the part through which the force is exerted to do the circular movement.

- The movement should be slow and harmonious.

- Exert light force rather than heavy force; exert force slowly rather than quickly.

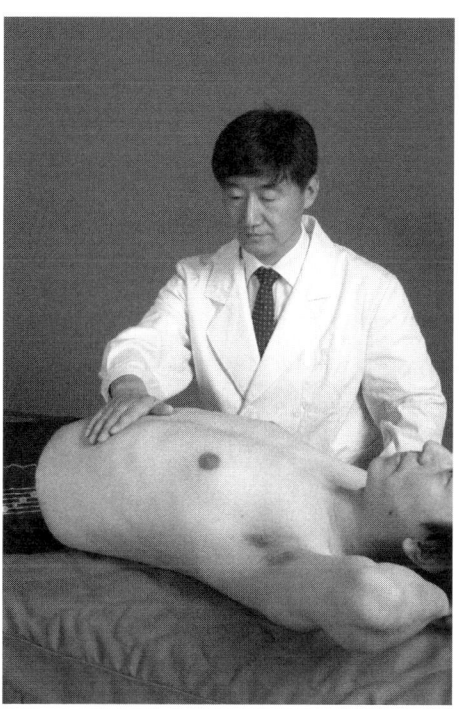

FUNCTION

Regulate gastrointestinal function, prevent ankylenteron (intestinal adhesion) after surgery. Rubbing can dredge the abdomen if it is done in a clockwise direction. It can reduce abnormal movements of the bowel if it is done in a counter-clockwise direction.

Figure 2.32 Rubbing the abdomen

NOTE

Exert light force rather than heavy force; exert force slowly rather than quickly.

Pushing outwards across the forehead

METHOD

Place the radial aspect of the distal phalanx of the thumbs on the middle point of forehead. Push from the midline of the forehead outwards to either side (Figure 2.33).

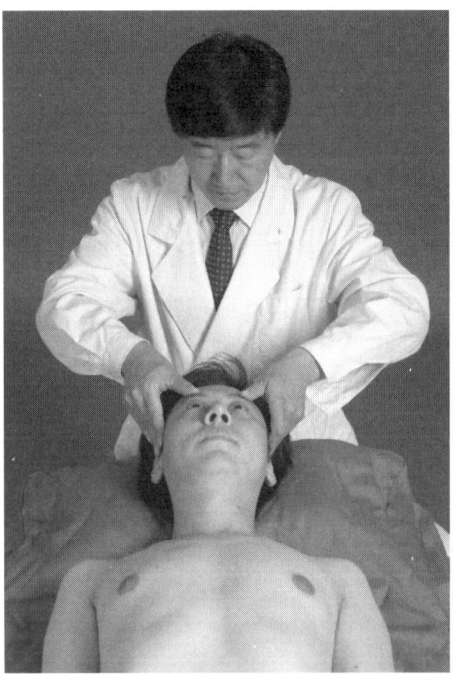

Figure 2.33 Pushing outwards across the forehead

THE MOVEMENT

• Exert light force rather than heavy force; exert force slowly rather than quickly.

• Pressing and kneading on acupoints can be used when pushing across them.

FUNCTION

Tranquilizing and allaying excitement.

NOTE

A certain amount of lubricant can be used in order to protect the patient's skin if it is dry.

Grasping manipulation

METHOD

Put the thumb on the opposite side of the four fingers so that the hand is pincer-shaped; exert opposing forces, generated by flexing and extending the metacarpophalangeal joints. Pinch and grasp the area to be treated. Grasping manipulation is done by alternately pinching, lifting, and letting go (Figure 2.34).

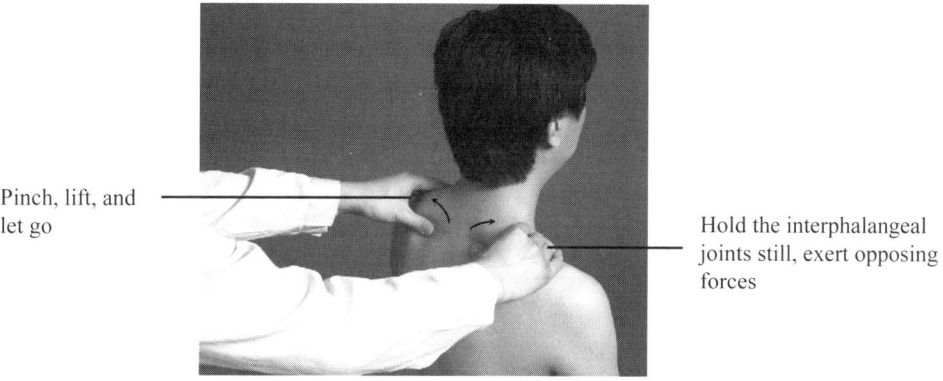

Pinch, lift, and let go

Hold the interphalangeal joints still, exert opposing forces

Figure 2.34 Grasping manipulation

THE MOVEMENT

- Relax the forearm, make the palm hollow.
- The direction of pinching and grasping should be perpendicular to the direction of the muscle belly.
- The movement should be continuous.
- Use light force at first and harder force later; no sudden impact.
- The force generated by movement of the metacarpophalangeal joints is the main motive power in pinching and grasping the muscle belly. There should be no movement of the interphalangeal joints.

FUNCTION

This technique affects the muscle layer. It has the function of releasing muscle spasm, enhancing excitation of the muscle, and relieving fatigue.

NOTE

There should be no movement of the interphalangeal joints during the grasping manipulation. Movement of interphalangeal joints would create a sense of being clutched, and this would impair relaxation.

This technique is gentle, and can be used widely, on male and female, old people and children, no matter whether the body is deficient or strong.

Percussing with the sides of the hands

METHOD

Stretch out the five fingers naturally, extend the wrist, and exert force through the ulnar side of the hand (including the fifth finger and hypothenar), percussing the body elastically and rhythmically with both hands alternately (Figure 2.35); or put the palms together, and percuss the area to be treated with both hands at once.

THE MOVEMENT

- Relax the elbow and wrist, and percuss elastically.
- The manipulation should be performed rhythmically, for the patient to feel relaxed and comfortable.

FUNCTION

This technique affects the muscle layer. It releases muscle spasm by vibration, and relieves muscle fatigue. It is commonly used at the end of a treatment.

NOTE

This technique is not suitable for using on the nape and occiput for too long.

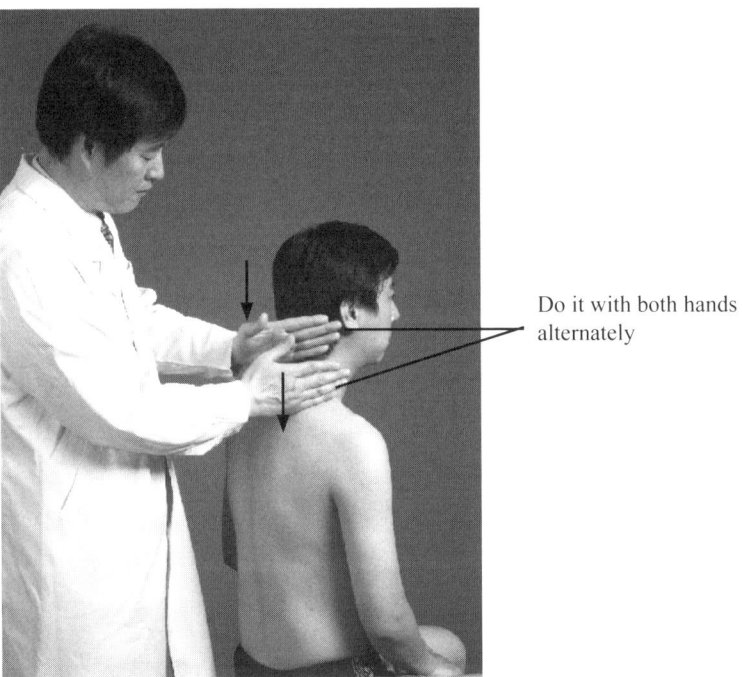

Do it with both hands alternately

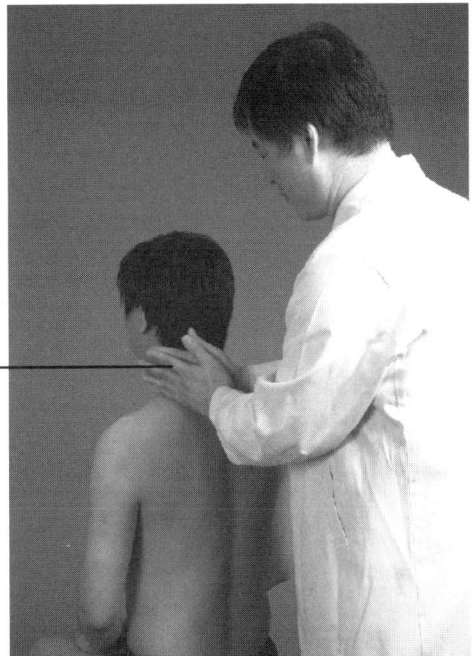

Do it with both hands together ———————

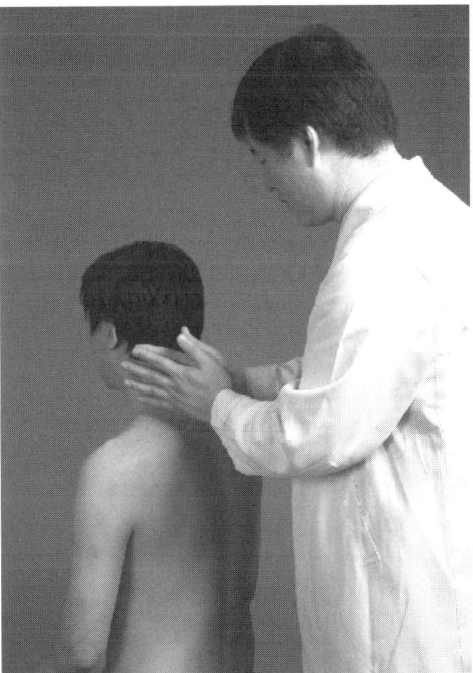

Figure 2.35 Lateral-palm percussing manipulation

Digital acupoint pressure

METHOD

Pressing on a point is called 'digital-pressing manipulation,' or 'digital acupoint pressure.' In digital acupoint pressure, the acupoint can be pressed by the thumb, index finger, or the index finger and middle finger together. It can be performed with one or both hands, or with two hands alternately (Figure 2.36).

THE MOVEMENT

The position and movement of the hand should be constant, to avoid injury to the fingers.

FUNCTION

This technique affects the deeper layer of tissue. While it is being done, the part to be treated should feel sore, numb, distending, heavy to the patient. It has the function of dredging the meridian passage, restoring the internal organs, regulating the movement of qi. It is usually used for easing pain, optimizing the function of internal organs. Make a concrete analysis and choose and coordinate acupoints according to the specific syndrome before applying this technique during treatment.

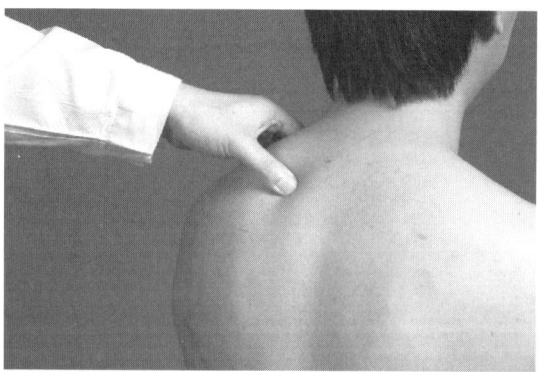

Figure 2.36 Digital acupoint pressure

NOTE

Take care with regard to both the doctor's fingers and the patient's skin when using digital-pressing manipulation.

The level of stimulus of this technique is high, and it takes effect rapidly.

Percussing with the fingertips

METHOD

Flex the fingers and thumbs of both hands, and exert force through the pads of the fingers, percussing the patient's calvaria elastically and rhythmically (Figure 2.37).

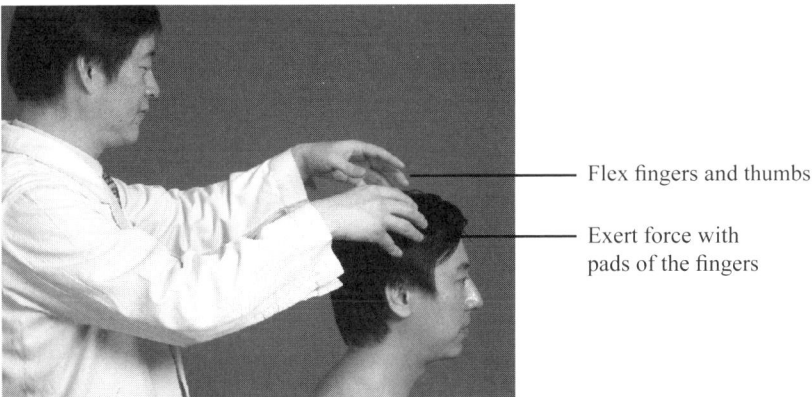

Flex fingers and thumbs

Exert force with pads of the fingers

Figure 2.37 Percussing with the fingertips

THE MOVEMENT

- Relax the wrist, flex and extend the elbow before bringing the wrist to sway freely, then percuss elastically.
- Work rhythmically, so that the patient feels relaxed and comfortable.
- If the fingertip percussing is done with both hands, the recommendation is to percuss both sides of the calvaria simultaneously. Percussing with two hands alternately can only be done on the calvaria.

FUNCTION

This technique affects the scalp and the layer beneath the scalp. It can be used to induce resuscitation and restore consciousness, to improve blood circulation in the scalp, and is mainly used at the end of a treatment.

NOTE

The skin should be protected.

When the technique is done correctly, the patient will feel relaxed and comfortable. It is one that people accept readily.

Wiping manipulation

METHOD

The patient lies on his back. The doctor sits at the head of the bed and applies the entire surface of both thumbs to EX-HN-3 Yintang; all four fingers of both hands are placed on the lateral sides of the head. Move the proximal part of the thumb initially, and slide the distal part of the thumb to DU-24 Shenting (Figure 2.38).

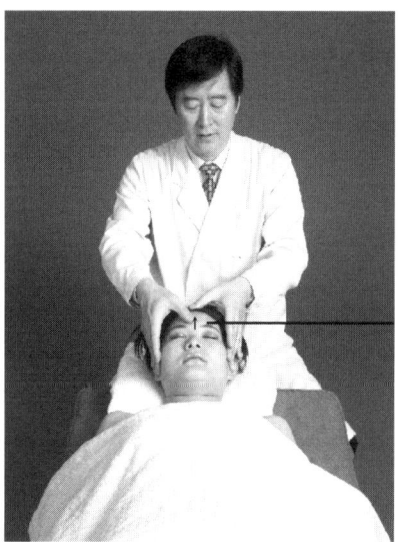

From EX-HN-3 Yintang to DU-24 Shenting, with both thumbs alternately

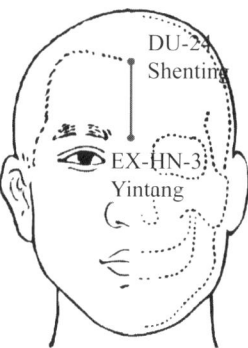

Figure 2.38 Wiping manipulation

THE MOVEMENT

- Exert light force rather than heavy force; exert force slowly rather than quickly.

- Work by moving the proximal part of the thumb first, and then the distal part of the thumb.

- The force, speed, and position of the two hands should be symmetrical.

FUNCTION

The stimulus is gentle and shallow, affecting the skin and hypodermic layer, but not the deeper layer of subcutaneous tissue. It has the function of tranquilizing and allaying excitement. This technique can be applied to the vertebral artery type of cervical spondylosis.

NOTE

Don't press the local part when doing this technique.

The stimulus of this technique is low, light, and gentle.

Combing hair

METHOD

The patient lies on his back. The doctor sits at the head of the bed, flexes the fingers and thumbs of both hands, places them on either side of the head, and combs the hair from the front of the head to the back (Figure 2.39).

THE MOVEMENT

Do the combing hair movement from the front of the head to the back quickly and lightly.

FUNCTION

It affects the scalp and the layer beneath. It has the function of tranquilizing and allaying excitement, and can be applied to the vertebral artery type of cervical spondylosis.

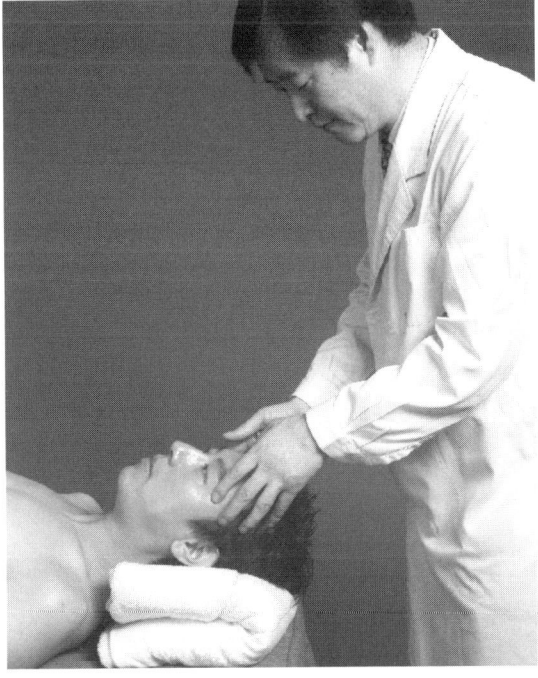

Figure 2.39 Combing hair

Twisting the fingers

METHOD

Twist and knead the part to be treated with the entire surface of the thumb and the radial side of the index finger, with opposing forces, and rapidly. This technique is applied to the fingers (Figure 2.40) and ear.

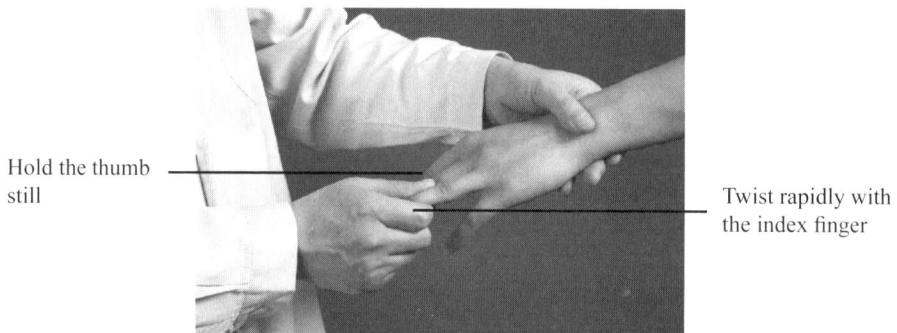

Hold the thumb still

Twist rapidly with the index finger

Figure 2.40 Finger-twisting manipulation

THE MOVEMENT

- Twist quickly, move slowly.
- Twisting is done by using the index finger first, and then the thumb.
- The movement should be continuous.

FUNCTION

The finger-twisting manipulation is applied mainly to the fingers and the ear. It affects only the skin and the subcutaneous layer. When the finger-twisting manipulation is applied to both sides of the finger, it has the function of dredging dermal parts, and is used to treat cervical spondylotic radiculopathy. When applied to the ear, it is used mainly to benefit the mind, and to treat cervical spondylotic radiculopathy.

NOTE

Twist quickly, move slowly.
   The stimulus of this technique is gentle and tender.

To-and-fro rubbing manipulation

METHOD

With the patient seated, the doctor stands behind him and places one hand on the affected shoulder. Keeping the fingers of the other hand together, exert force on the palm of the hand and make the force act on the shoulder, rubbing rapidly to-and-fro (Figure 2.41).

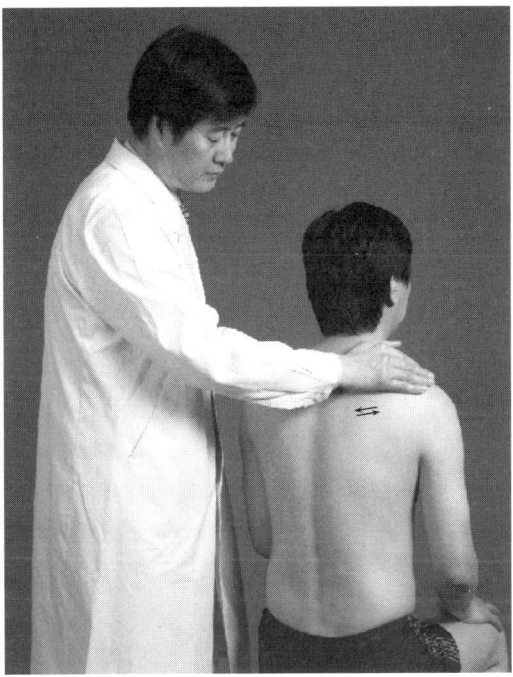

Figure 2.41 To-and-fro rubbing manipulation

THE MOVEMENT

- Rub to-and-fro in a straight line; the line should not deviate.
- The part of the hand on which the force is exerted should be closely connected with the skin; the pressure should be moderate.
- The movement should be continuous, the rapidity of the movement should be even and high, and the length of the to-and-fro movement should be as great as possible.

FUNCTION

The manipulation affects first the superficial layer, then the deeper layer. It has the effect of warming and dredging meridians. It is used to treat cold diseases.

The effect of the manipulation is that the heat reaches first the superficial layer, then the deeper layer, which is called 'penetrating heat.'

NOTE

- The part to be treated is best left uncovered.

- Use a suitable amount of lubricant on the part to be treated – for example, massage lotion, oil of turpentine.

- This technique is used mainly at the end of a treatment.

- When doing this manipulation, the doctor should breathe naturally, without holding the breath.

Although the force generated by this technique is light, the heat generated by it can penetrate to deeper tissues, which is called 'penetrating heat.'

Stretching the brachial plexus

METHOD

The patient sits, and the doctor stands behind them on the affected side. The doctor presses his abdomen against the patient's back and lifts the patient's arm, with the elbow straight, the wrist dorsiflexed, and the fingers pointing to the posterior lateral side (Figure 2.42).

THE MOVEMENT

It is best to raise the affected arm at an angle of 135°.

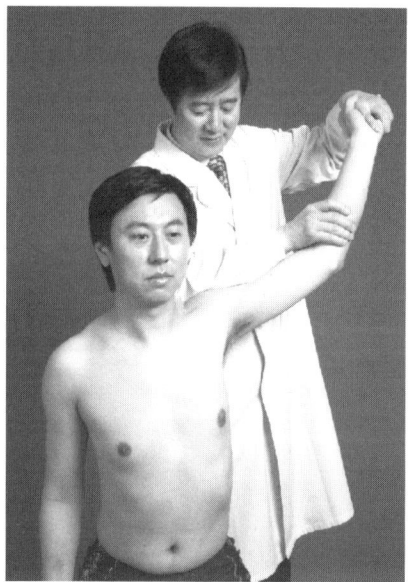

FUNCTION

This technique can be used to prevent adhesion of the nerve root, or separate adhesion of the nerve root, and can be used to great effect to reduce numbness and pain in the upper limbs.

NOTE

The doctor should press his abdomen against the patient's back.

Figure 2.42 Stretching the brachial plexus

Pulling manipulation of the rotated and localized neck

METHOD

We will use the example of right deviation of a spinous process. The patient sits. The doctor stands behind the patient on the patient's right side, and presses his left thumb against the right side of the affected spinous process. He bends the patient's head to the required angle, and when the spinous process of the affected vertebra starts to move, he bends the head to the left, before rotating the patient's face as far as possible to the right. The doctor then supports the patient's lower jaw with his right hand and, once the patient is relaxed, suddenly performs a small, rapid, and controlled thrust, with the left thumb simultaneously pushing the affected spinous process to the left. At this point the sound of a slight click or snap indicates a successful outcome (Figure 2.43). The doctor can also use his elbow to support the patient's lower jaw (Figure 2.44).

THE MOVEMENT

- Orientation should be precise: bend the head forward until the spinous process of the affected vertebra moves, then bend the head laterally as far as possible and rotate as far as possible.

- The force should be stable, precise, deft: a small, rapid controlled thrust, with the thumb pushing the affected spinous process to the right/left (as appropriate).

- The thrust should be exerted when the head is rotated to the maximum extent possible.

FUNCTION

This technique is used to make the cervical spine rotate on its vertical axis.

NOTE

- Make the patient fully relax before pulling.

- Orientation should be precise; don't try too hard to obtain the snapping sound.

- This manipulation should either be used with caution, or else excluded, when treating patients with the vertebral artery type of cervical spondylosis, cervical spondylotic myelopathy, serious heart and lung problems, and various types of bone disease such as osteonosus, and rachiterata.

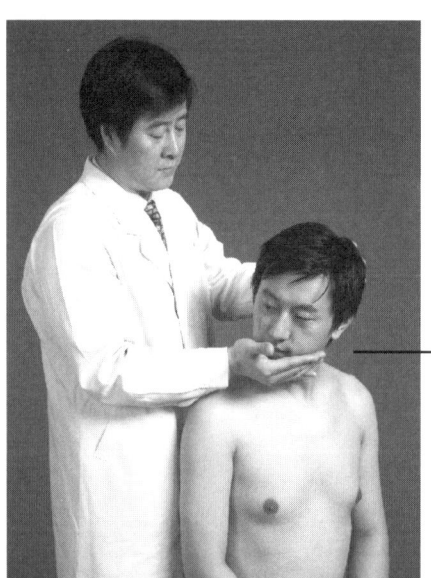

Bend head forward until the spinous process of the affected vertebra moves, then bend the head laterally as far as possible, rotate as far as possible

Figure 2.43 Pulling manipulation of the rotated and localized neck (1)

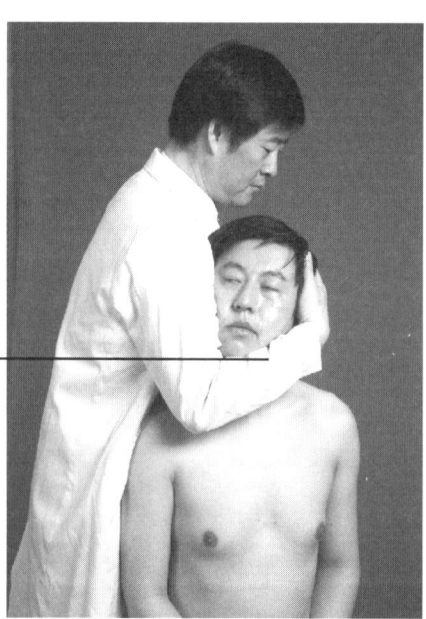

The doctor performs a small, rapid, and controlled thrust

Figure 2.44 Pulling manipulation of the rotated and localized neck (2)

Lateral pulling manipulation of the neck

METHOD

We will use the example of restricted movement when bending the neck to the left. The doctor stands on the right side of the patient. He presses his left elbow against the patient's right shoulder; his left hand hooks around the patient's nape from behind the head, and his right hand is placed on the right side of the head (above the right ear). First, bend the patient's head to the left to the maximum extent possible, then exert a sudden force, increasing the lateral bending further by an angle of 5–10°, and with that release both hands (Figure 2.45).

THE MOVEMENT

Exert a sudden force once the head is bent to the maximum extent possible, to increase the angle of lateral bending. A sudden force should be momentary, singular, and direct (namely, exert the force directly when the head is bent to the maximum extent).

FUNCTION

Used to restore the function of bending the neck laterally.

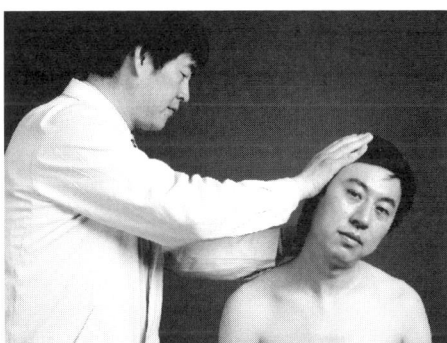

Bend to the side to the maximum extent possible, then exert a sudden force —

Fix —

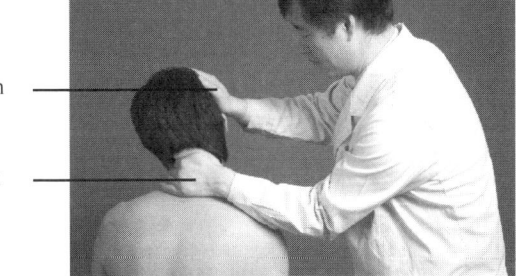

Figure 2.45 Lateral pulling manipulation of the neck

NOTE

Taking the example of restricted movement when bending the neck to the right: this technique is applicable if pain is located on the left side, but is inapplicable if the pain is located on the right side.

Holding and stretching the cervical spine

METHOD

The patient sits on a low stool, with both legs extended forwards, and both hands on his thighs. The doctor stands on the posterior lateral side of the patient. With one hand supporting the occiput, and the elbow of the other arm gripping the patient's lower jaw, he first stretches slowly upward, sustains the stretching force until the nape of the patient is relatively relaxed, and then exerts a sudden upward force, stretching the patient's cervical spine.

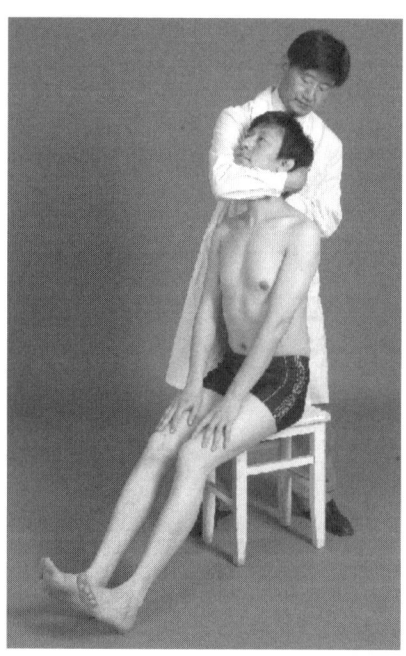

Figure 2.46 Holding and stretching the cervical spine

THE MOVEMENT

The key to success with this manipulation technique is to choose the right moment, when the patient is relaxed, and exert a sudden upward force while maintaining the force of traction.

FUNCTION

Apart from the above-mentioned functions, the technique of holding and stretching the cervical spine can also adjust the cervical intervertebral joints, and correct rotation on the frontal axis and sagittal axis of cervical vertebrae. It is used mainly to treat disturbance of cervical intervertebral joints when there is a sprain of the neck, or stiffness of the neck.

NOTE

When carrying out holding and stretching of the cervical spine, ensure that the patient is in the correct posture.

Rotating the neck

METHOD

- **Method 1:** The patient sits, with his neck relaxed. The doctor stands on the patient's posterior lateral side. Using one hand to support the occiput, and the elbow of the other arm to grip the patient's lower jaw, he slowly rotates the patient's neck, gradually increasing the range of rotation. Using the same method, he then rotates the patient's neck in the reverse direction (Figure 2.47).

- **Method 2:** The doctor stands behind the patient. Using both hands to support the head (thumbs placed at the rear of the head, fingers at the front to support the lower jaw), he presses the ulnar sides of his forearms against the patient's shoulders, and slowly rotates the neck with an upward stretch, gradually increasing the range of rotation (Figure 2.48).

THE MOVEMENT

- Rotate slowly, not quickly, otherwise the patient will experience dizziness.

- A wide range of rotation is inadvisable; keep rotation within a limited range.

- As he increases the range of rotation, the doctor moves from the patient's lateral side to the posterior side. The recommended direction of rotation is: inferior side – lateral side – superior side – doctor's side, with the lower jaw as the point of reference.

FUNCTION

This technique can increase the range of movement of the neck and is used mainly to treat cervical spondylosis, or a stiff neck.

NOTE

- Use this technique with caution when treating patients experiencing dizziness.

- High speed and wide range of rotation is inadvisable; keep rotation to a limited range.

- Ask patients to keep their eyes open during rotation, otherwise they may experience dizziness.

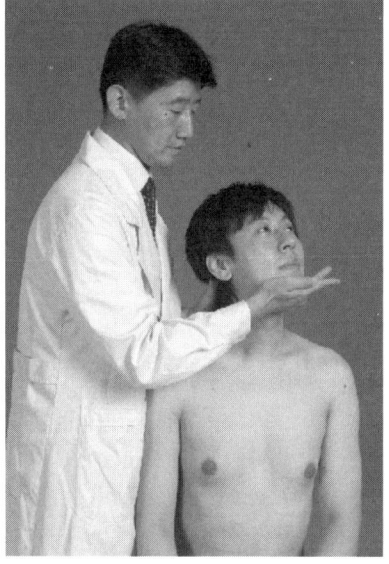

a

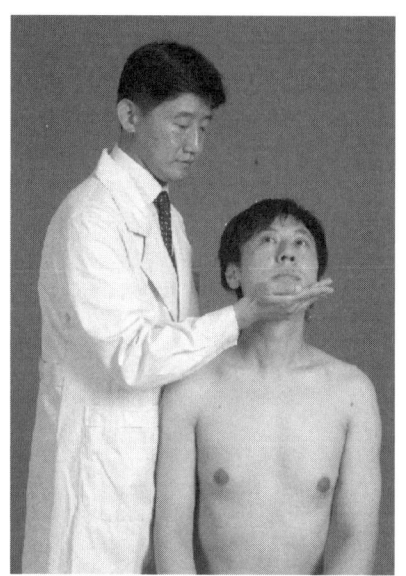

b

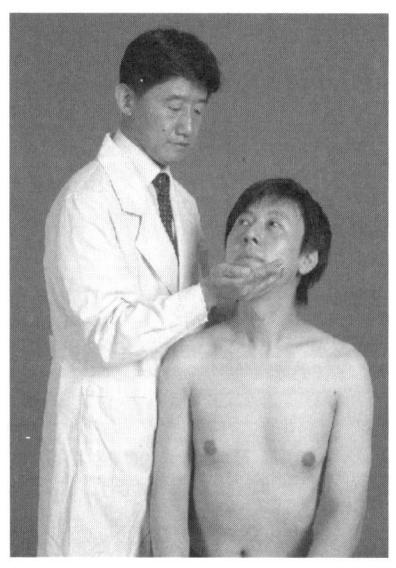

c

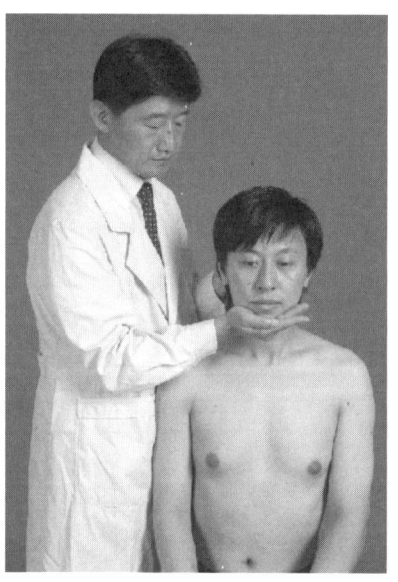

d

Figure 2.47 Rotation of the neck (method 1)

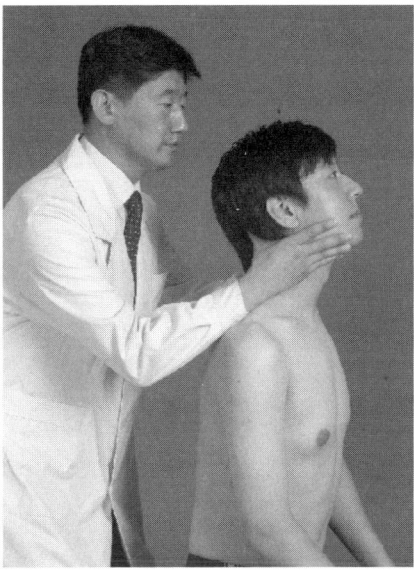

Figure 2.48 Rotation of the neck (method 2)

Traction of the cervical spine

METHOD

- **Traction of the cervical spine in the sitting position:** The patient sits. The doctor stands on the patient's posterior lateral side. Pressing his abdomen against the patient's back, with one hand supporting the occiput, and the elbow of the other arm gripping the patient's lower jaw, he stretches the patient's cervical spine in a backwards and upwards direction, slowly and repeatedly (Figure 2.49).

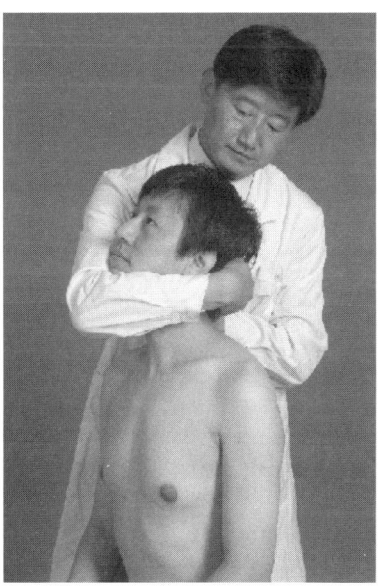

Figure 2.49 Traction of the cervical spine in the sitting position

- **Traction of the cervical spine in the lying position:** The patient lies down. The doctor uses one hand to support the occiput, places the other hand on the patient's lower jaw, and exerts force with both hands to stretch the patient's cervical spine (Figure 2.50).

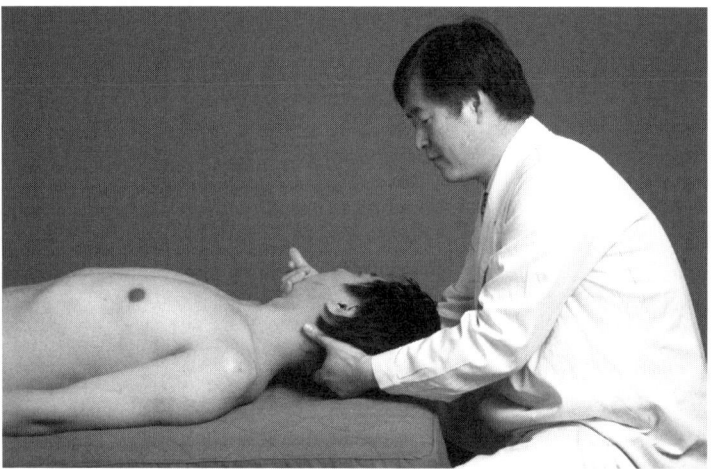

Figure 2.50 Traction of the cervical spine in the lying position

THE MOVEMENT

- The doctor stands on the patient's posterior lateral side.
- The patient bends his head backward to an angle of around 30° while being stretched.
- The doctor exerts force with both hands simultaneously.

FUNCTION

Traction of the cervical spine can increase the cervical intervertebral space and reduce pressure on the inner part of the intervertebral disk. It is used mainly to treat cervical spondylosis.

NOTE

It is the lower jaw, not the neck, that is gripped by the elbow, no matter which type of traction is used.

Chapter *3*

Massage Therapy Treatment for Cervical Spondylosis

Section I Massage Therapy Treatment for Cervical Spondylosis

1. Loosening tendons by pressing and kneading

The initial step of treatment is to loosen tendons, that is to say, to relax the muscles of nape. The following manipulations can be applied to the treatment, according to the practical condition and the practitioner's level of mastery. The manipulations should be performed on the Governor Vessel, Jiaji, the Gallbladder Meridian of Foot-Shaoyang, and the Sanjiao meridian of Hand-Shaoyang in the region of the occiput, nape, shoulder, and back.

- *The first step of treatment* is a pushing manipulation with one finger on the nape (Figure 3.1). The manipulation should be applied to the occiput, nape, and shoulder from the upper region to the lower region, from the medial region to the lateral regions, and from the normal side to the affected side. The force of manipulation should be light at first, and then heavy. The force of manipulation reaches first the superficial layer, and then the deeper layer, in order to fully relax these regions.

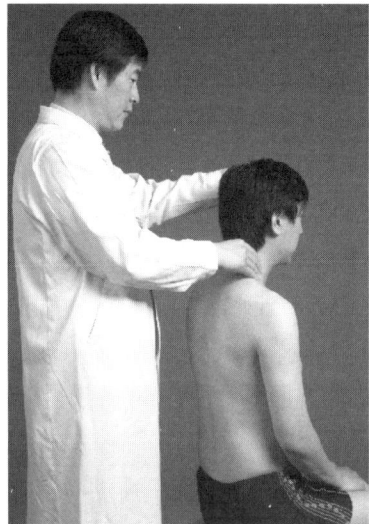
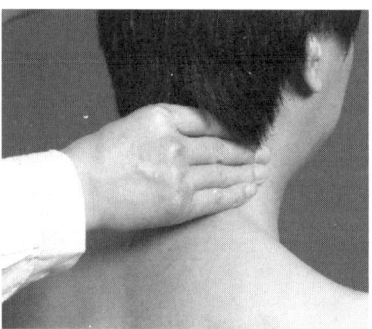

Figure 3.1 Pushing manipulation with one finger on the nape

- *The second step of treatment* is a grasping manipulation (Figure 3.2). The force of manipulation should be deep and steady. It is performed first to relax the muscles of the superficial layer on the lateral sides of the nape, then to relax the muscles of the deeper layer. Avoid lifting the grasped tissue excessively, otherwise the patient will feel as if he is being strangled. Grasping and kneading techniques can be used in combination.

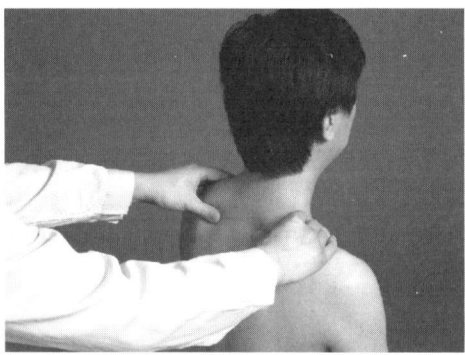
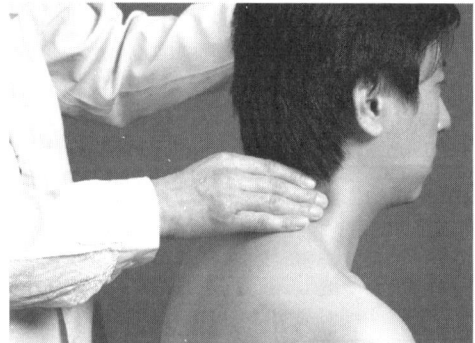

Figure 3.2 Grasping manipulation

- *The third step of treatment* is a rolling manipulation on the shoulder (Figure 3.3). The doctor asks the patient to sit with his head bent to the *normal* side, to thoroughly expose the affected side when rolling on the nape; and to sit with his head bent to the *affected* side to relax the muscles when rolling on the shoulder. Lateral rolling is suitable for the nape and shoulder. Vertical rolling is suitable for the junction of the nape and shoulders and on the back.

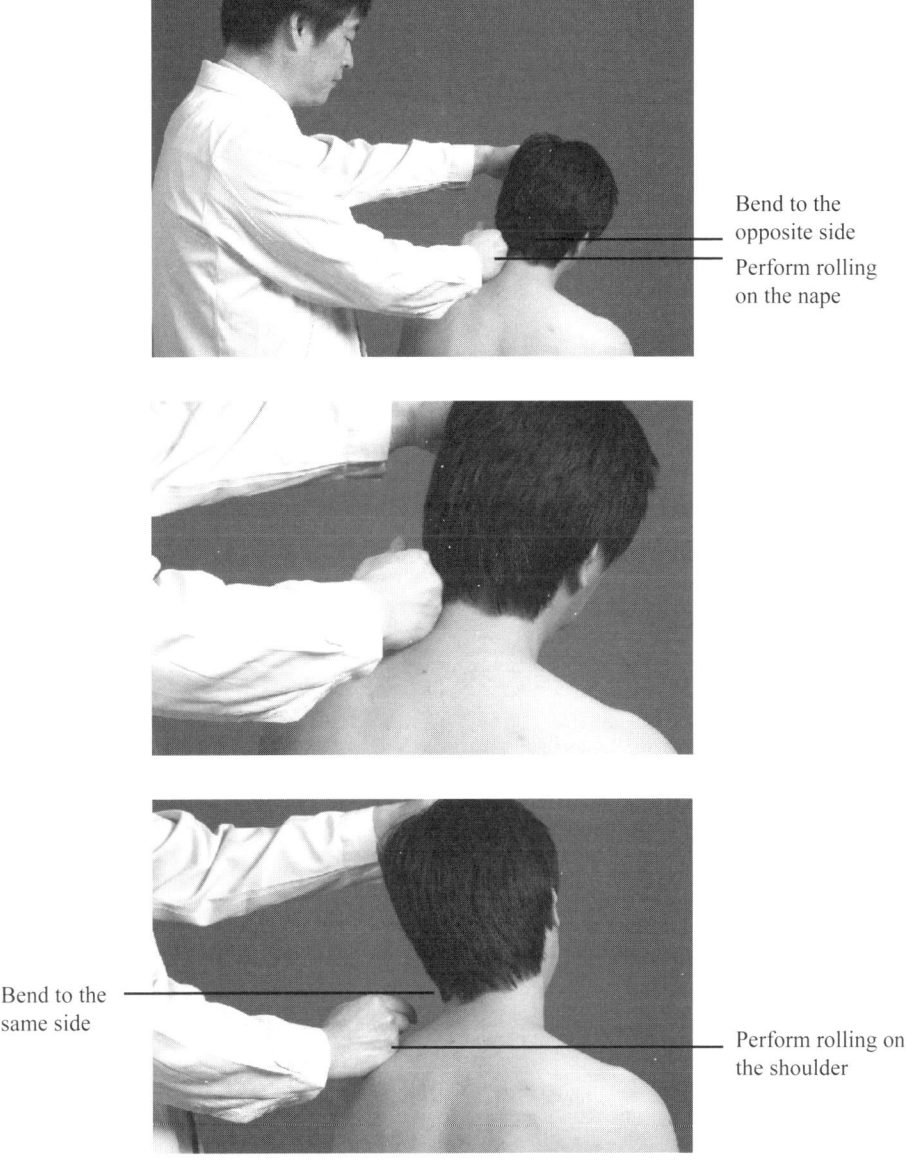

Figure 3.3 Rolling manipulation on the shoulder

- *The fourth step of treatment* involves kneading with the thumb or four fingers on the muscles of both sides of the nape (Figure 3.4). It is performed from the upper region to the lower region of the nape, first to relax the muscles of the superficial layer, then to relax the muscles of the deeper layer.

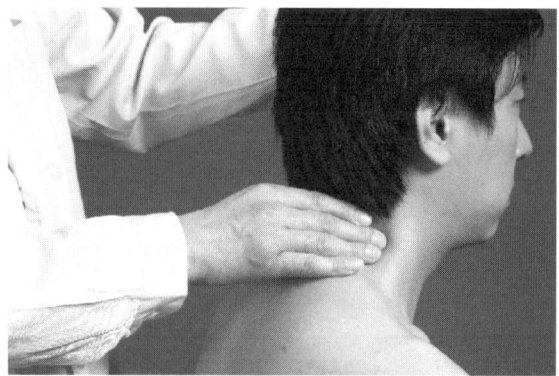

Figure 3.4 Kneading with finger manipulation

2. Digital pressing and kneading of pain spots

Digital pressing, kneading, and plucking on pain spots are the foundation of work on the nape and shoulders (Figure 3.5). These techniques are used to ease pain, relieve spasm, and free adhesion.

This technique can be combined with pressing and kneading for loosening tendons, depending on the condition, in order to improve the effect of manipulation.

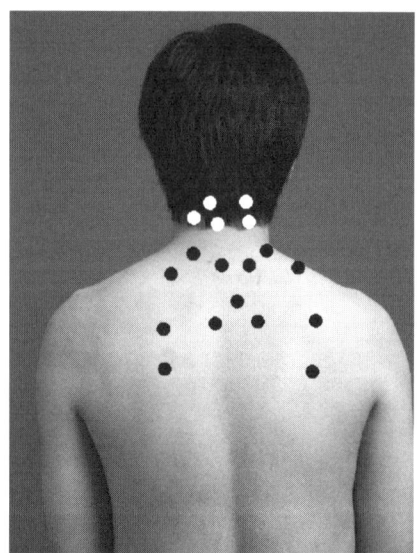

Figure 3.5 Common pain spots of cervical spondylosis

3. Treatment according to the different types of cervical spondylosis

STIFF NECK TYPE OF CERVICAL SPONDYLOSIS

The key is to use relaxing manipulation on the nape and shoulder.

CERVICAL SPONDYLOTIC RADICULOPATHY

Use digital pressing, kneading, and plucking on the appropriate acupoints. The purpose is to dredge the meridian passage, regulate and activate qi and blood, and treat numbness and pain in the fingers.

ST-12 Quepen

Location: At the centre of the supraclavicular fossa, 4 cun lateral to the anterior midline (Figure 3.6).

Indications: Pain and numbness in the upper arm.

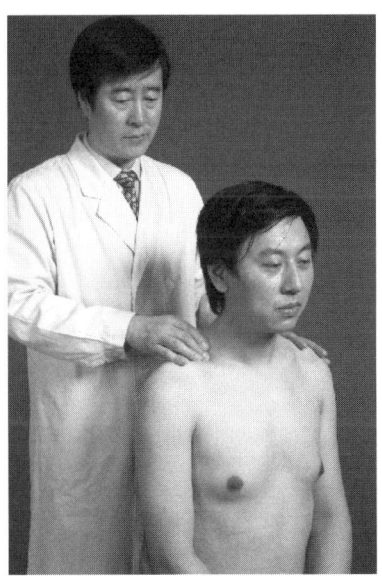 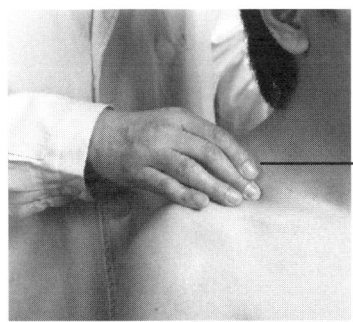

Exert force by using the middle finger, from the front to the rear

Figure 3.6 Digital pressing on ST-12 Quepen

SI-15 Jianzhongshu

Location: On the back, below the spinous process of the seventh cervical vertebra, 2 cun lateral to the posterior midline (Figure 3.7).

Indications: Pain in the shoulder and back.

SI-14 Jianwaishu

Location: On the back, below the spinous process of the first thoracic vertebra, 3 cun lateral to the posterior midline (Figure 3.7).

Indications: Pain in the shoulder and back.

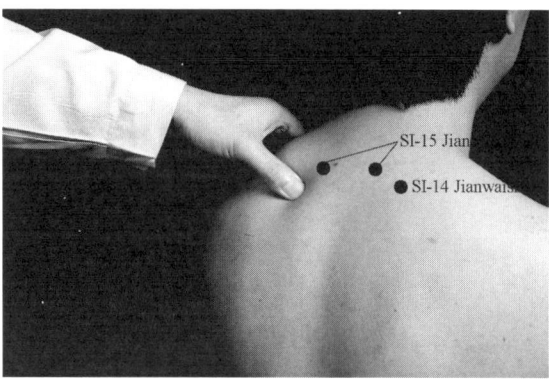

Figure 3.7 Digital pressing on SI-15 Jianzhongshu and SI-14 Jianwaishu

GB-21 Jianjing

Location: On the scapula, at the midpoint of the line connecting the spinous process of C7 and the lateral point of the acromion (Figure 3.8).

Indications: Pain in the shoulder and neck.

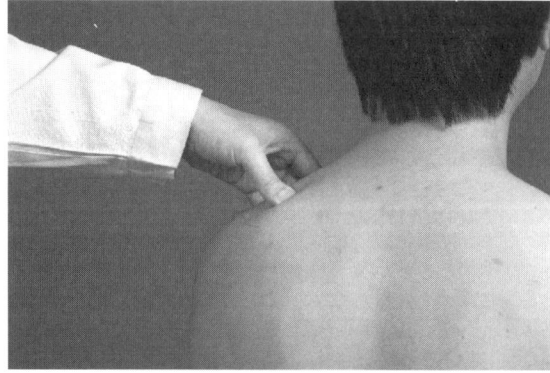

Figure 3.8 Digital pressing on GB-21 Jianjing

SI-11 Tianzong

Location: On the scapula, in the depression of the centre of the subscapular fossa, and level with the fourth thoracic vertebra (Figure 3.9).

Indications: Shoulder and back pain, pain in the medial part of the upper arm.

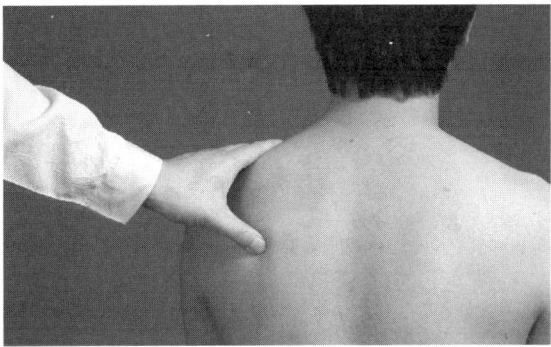

Figure 3.9 Digital pressing on SI-11 Tianzong

SI-9 Jianzhen

Location: Posterior and inferior to the shoulder joint, 1 cun above the posterior end of the axillary fold with the arm adducted (Figure 3.10).

Indications: Pain in the medial part of the upper arm, pain and numbness in the little finger.

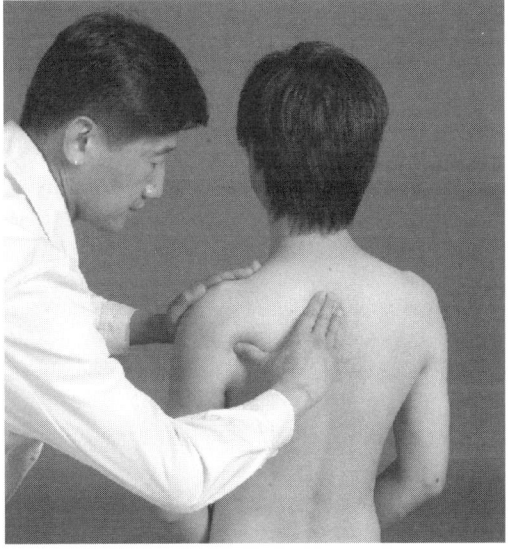

Figure 3.10 Digital pressing on SI-9 Jianzhen

HT-1 Jiquan

Location: At the apex of the axillary fossa, where the pulsation of the axillary artery is palpable (Figure 3.11).

Indications: Pain and numbness in the upper arm.

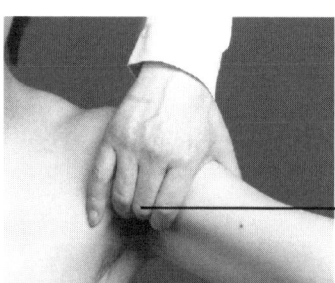

Exert force along the posterior border of deltoid, from the front to the rear

Figure 3.11 Digital pressing on HT-1 Jiquan

LI-14 Binao

Location: On the lateral side of the arm, at the insertion of the deltoid muscle and on the line connecting LI-11 Quchi and LI-15 Jianyu, 7 cun above LI-11 Quchi (Figure 3.12).

Indications: Pain or numbness in the part of the hand between the thumb and the index finger.

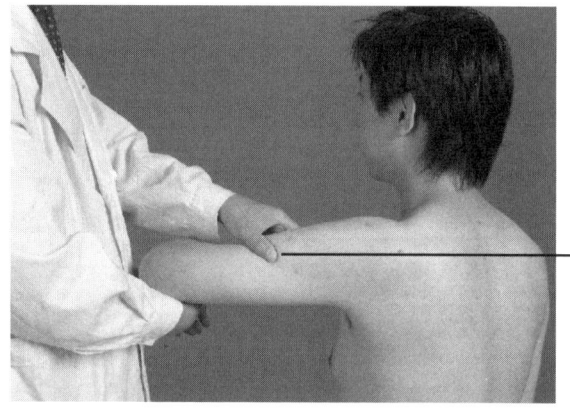

Exert force along the posterior border of the deltoid, from the front to the rear

Figure 3.12 Digital pressing on LI-14 Binao

LI-11 Quchi

Location: With the elbow flexed, at the lateral end of the cubital crease, at the midpoint of the line connecting LU-5 Chize and external humeral epicondyle (Figure 3.13).

Indications: Pain on the lateral side of the forearm.

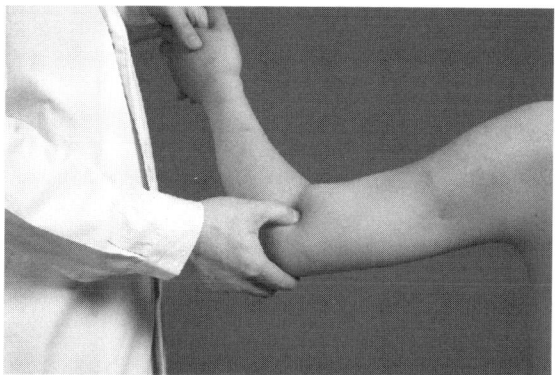

Figure 3.13 Digital pressing on LI-11 Quchi

LI-10 Shousanli

Location: On the radial side of the dorsal surface of the forearm and 2 cun below the cubital crease, on the line connecting LI-5 Yangxi and LI-11 Quchi (Figure 3.14).

Indications: Pain on the lateral side of the forearm and the back of the hand.

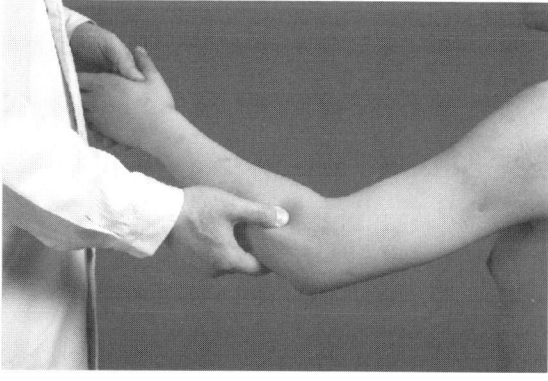

Figure 3.14 Digital pressing on LI-10 Shousanli

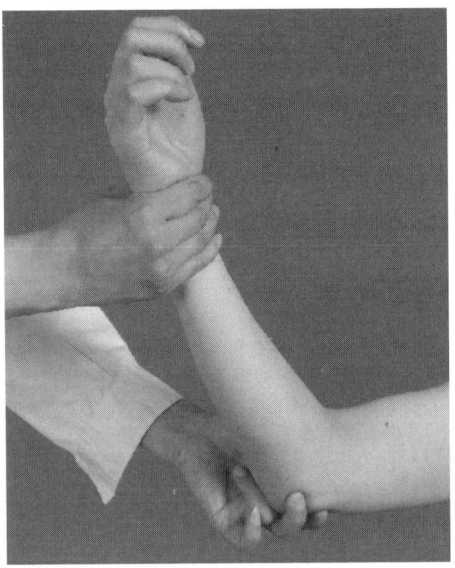

Figure 3.15 Digital pressing on SI-8 Xiaohai

SI-8 Xiaohai

Location: On the medial side of the elbow, in the depression between the olecranon of the ulna and the medial epicondyle of the humerus (Figure 3.15).

Indications: Pain in the forearm and medial side of the hand.

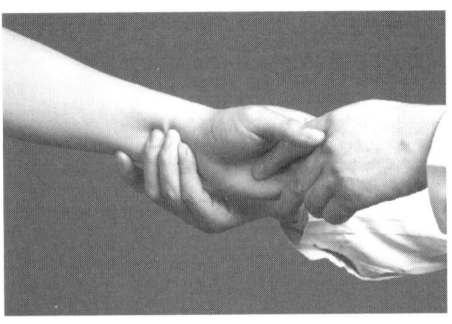

Figure 3.16 Digital pressing on PC-6 Neiguan

PC-6 Neiguan

Location: On the palmar side of the forearm, 2 cun above the crease of the wrist, between the tendon of palmaris longus and the tendon of flexor carpi radialis (Figure 3.16).

Indications: Pain, numbness, painful swelling of the palm.

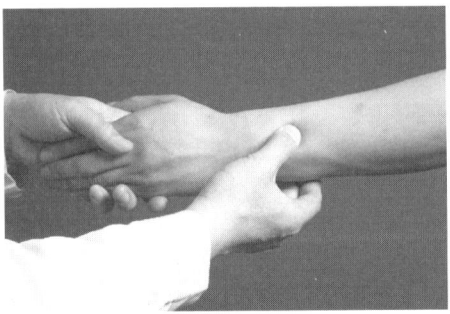

Figure 3.17 Digital pressing on TE-5 Waiguan

TE-5 Waiguan

Location: On the dorsal side of the forearm, 2 cun proximal to the dorsal crease of the wrist, on the central point of the space between the radius and ulna (Figure 3.17).

Indications: Pain on the back of the hand.

LI-4 Hegu

Location: On the dorsum of the hand, between the first and second metacarpal bones, and on the radial side of the midpoint of the second metacarpal bone (Figure 3.18).

Indications: Pain and numbness in the part of the hand between the thumb and the index finger, and in the index finger and thumb.

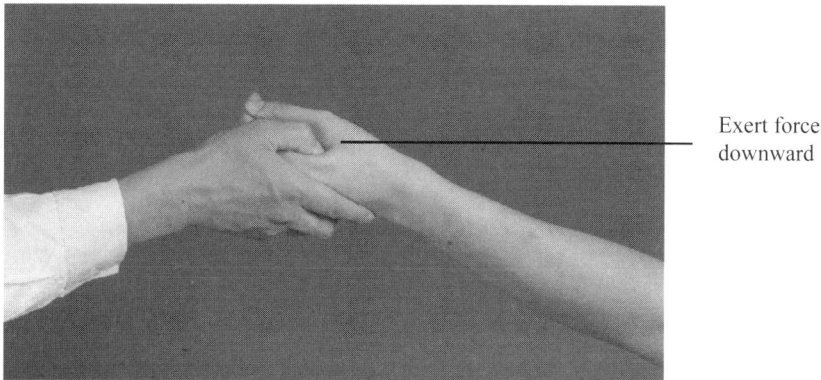

Exert force downward

Figure 3.18 Digital pressing on LI-4 Hegu

SI-3 Houxi

Location: At the junction of the red and white skin along the ulnar border of the hand, at the ulnar end of the distal palmar crease, proximal to the fifth metacarpophalangeal joint when a hollow fist is made (Figure 3.19).

Indications: Pain and numbness in the little finger and the ulnar side of palm.

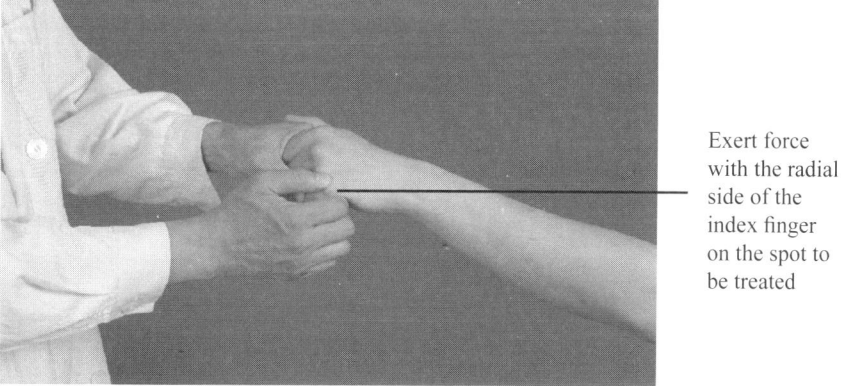

Exert force with the radial side of the index finger on the spot to be treated

Figure 3.19 Digital pressing on SI-3 Houxi

In addition to the above, the following techniques may be used in treating cervical spondylosis radiculopathy:

- twisting the fingers (see page 70)
- stretching the brachial plexus (see page 72).

VERTEBRAL ARTERY TYPE OF CERVICAL SPONDYLOSIS

Use the wiping manipulation described on p.68, and also the technique of pushing outwards across the forehead, described on p.62.

Press and knead acupoints EX-HN-5 Taiyang, ST-8 Touwei, SJ-20 Jiaosun, DU-20 Baihui, EX-HN-1 Sishencong.

EX-HN-5 Taiyang

Location: On the head, between the lateral end of the eyebrow and the outer canthus, in the depression one finger breadth behind them (Figure 3.20).

Indications: Dizziness, headache.

ST-8 Touwei

Location: On the head, 0.5 cun above the anterior hairline at the corner of the forenead, and 4.5 cun lateral to the midline of the head (Figure 3.21).

Indications: Splitting headache.

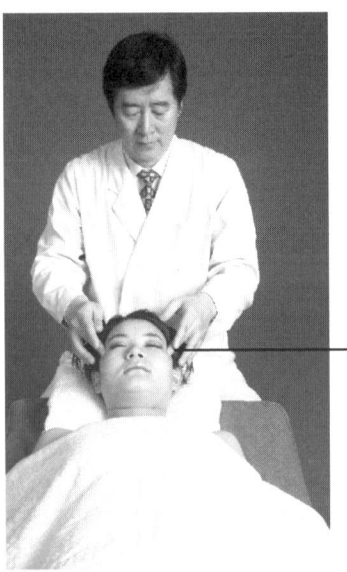

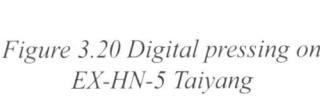

The force of the digital pressing and kneading should not exceed the patient's level of tolerance

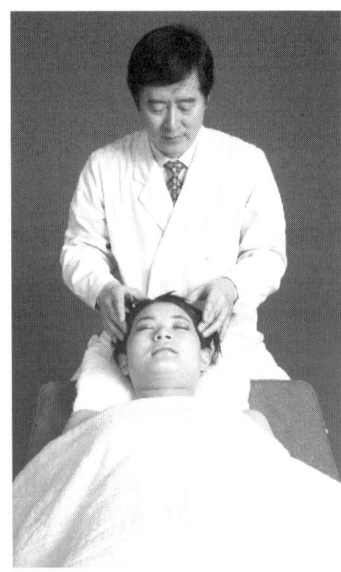

Figure 3.20 Digital pressing on EX-HN-5 Taiyang

Figure 3.21 Digital pressing on ST-8 Touwei

SJ-20 Jiaosun

Location: On the head, above the ear apex, within the hairline (Figure 3.22).

Indications: Splitting headache.

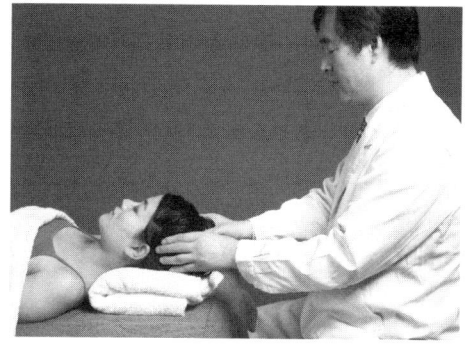

Figure 3.22 Digital pressing on SJ-20 Jiaosun

DU-20 Baihui

Location: On the head, 5 cun directly above the midpoint of the anterior hairline (Figure 3.23).

Indications: Headache, dizziness, splitting headache.

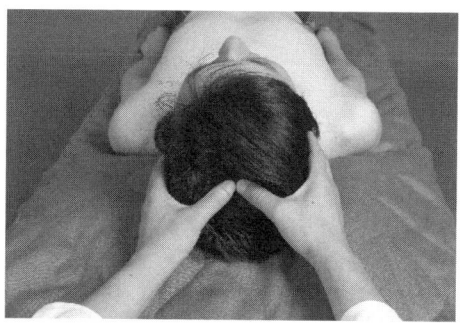

Figure 3.23 Digital pressing on DU-20 Baihui

EX-HN-1 Sishencong

Location: On the head, 1 cun anterior, posterior, and lateral to DU-20 Baihui (four acupoints altogether; Figure 3.24).

Indications: Headache, dizziness, splitting headache.

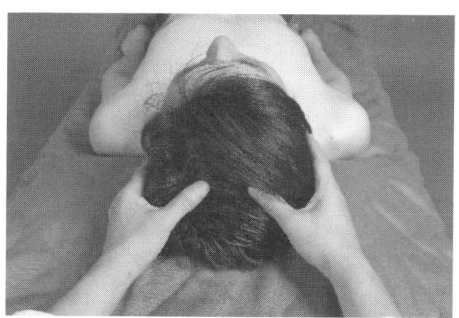 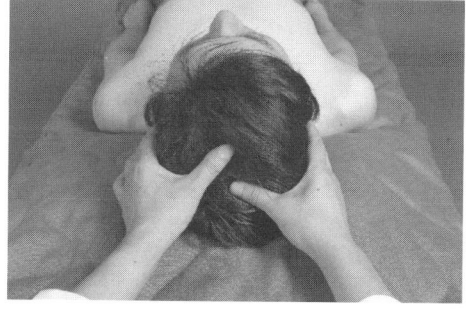

Figure 3.24 Digital pressing on EX-HN-1 Sishencong

CERVICAL SPONDYLOTIC MYELOPATHY

Use digital pressing and kneading of acupoints. In addition to digital pressing and kneading of the nape and shoulder, and manipulations used on the upper limbs, the acupoints on the lower limbs should also be treated by digital pressing and kneading. This will dredge the meridians of the lower limbs, and promote the circulation of qi and blood, to treat numbness and weakness in the lower limbs. The following acupoints are commonly treated with digital pressing.

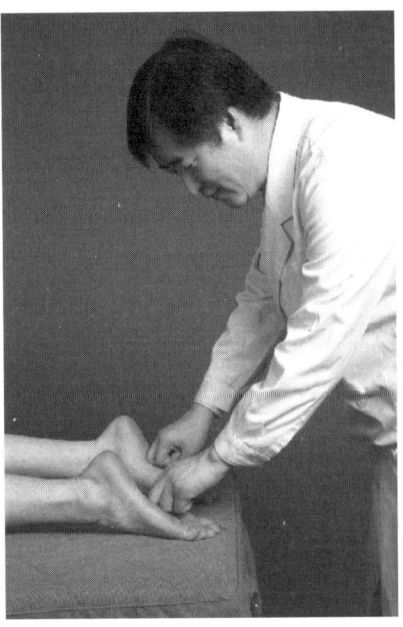

Figure 3.25 Digital pressing on
KI-1 Yongquan

KI-1 Yongquan

Location: On the thenar, in the depression appearing on the anterior part of the sole when the foot is in plantar flexion (Figure 3.25).

Indications: Numbness in toes, weakness of lower limbs.

BL-60 Kunlun

Location: Posterior to the lateral malleolus, in the depression between the tip of the external malleolus and the Achilles tendon (Figure 3.26).

Indications: Numbness in toes, pain in the thenar (sole of the foot).

KI-3 Taixi

Location: On the ankle, in the depression between the tip of the medial malleolus and the Achilles tendon (Figure 3.26).

Indications: Numbness in toes, pain in the thenar.

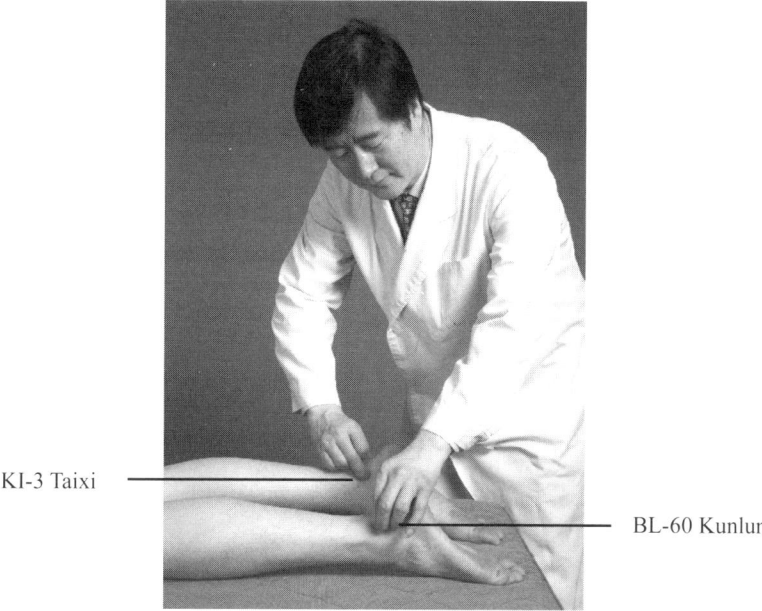

KI-3 Taixi

BL-60 Kunlun

Figure 3.26 Digital pressing on BL-60 Kunlun and KI-3 Taixi

GB-39 Xuanzhong

Location: On the lateral side of the shank, 3 cun above the tip of the external malleolus, on the anterior border of the fibula (Figure 3.27).

Indications: Numbness, pain, and weakness on the lateral side of the crus (lower leg).

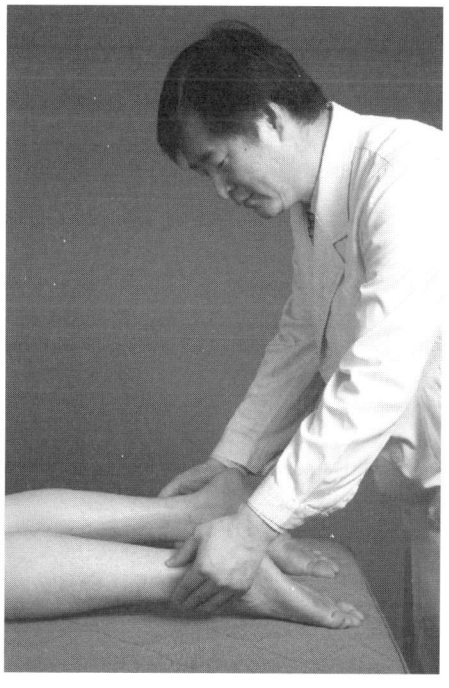

Figure 3.27 Digital pressing on GB-39 Xuanzhong

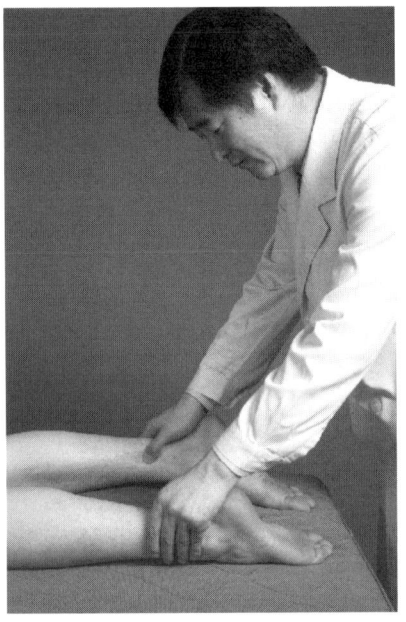

*Figure 3.28 Digital pressing on
SP-6 Sanyinjiao*

SP-6 Sanyinjiao

Location: On the medial side of the leg, 3 cun above the tip of the medial malleolus, posterior to the medial border of the tibia (Figure 3.28).

Indications: Pain, numbness, and weakness on the medial side of the crus and foot.

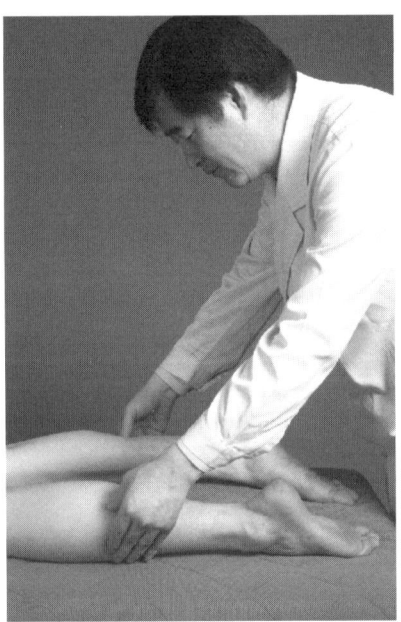

*Figure 3.29 Digital pressing on
BL-57 Chengshan*

BL-57 Chengshan

Location: On the posterior midline of the calf, between BL-40 Weizhong and BL-60 Kunlun, a pointed depression formed below the gastrocnemius muscle belly when the leg is stretched or the heel is lifted (Figure 3.29).

Indications: Numbness, pain, and weakness on the posterior side of the crus.

BL-40 Weizhong

Location: At the midpoint of the popliteal crease, between the tendon of the biceps femoris muscle and the semitendinosus muscle (Figure 3.30).

Indications: Numbness, pain, and weakness on the posterior side of the crus.

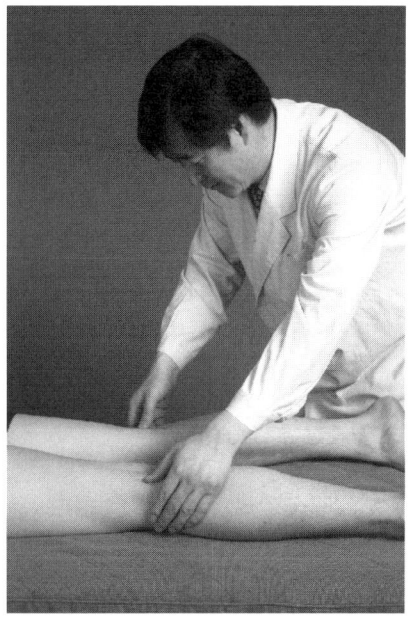

Figure 3.30 Digital pressing on BL-40 Weizhong

BL-39 Weiyang

Location: On the knee, on the lateral part of popliteal crease, medial to the tendon of the biceps femoris muscle (Figure 3.31).

Indications: Numbness, pain, and weakness on the lateral side of the crus.

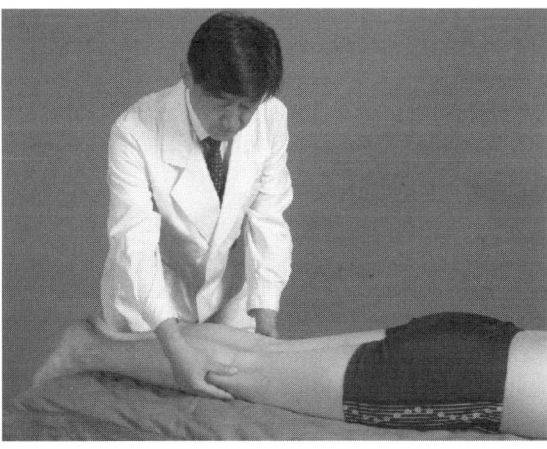

Figure 3.31 Digital pressing on BL-39 Weiyang

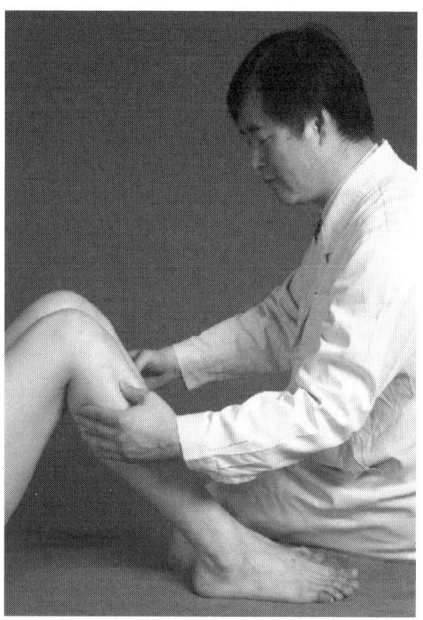

*Figure 3.32 Digital pressing on
GB-34 Yanglingquan*

GB-34 Yanglingquan

Location: On the lateral side of the shank, in a depression anterior and inferior to the head of the fibula (Figure 3.32).

Indications: Numbness, pain, and weakness on the lateral side of the crus.

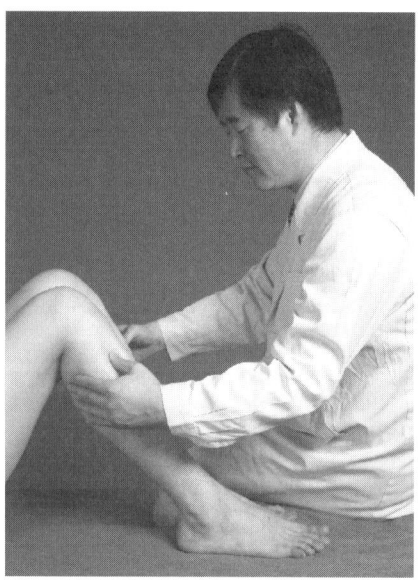

*Figure 3.33 Digital pressing on
ST-36 Zusanli*

ST-36 Zusanli

Location: On the anterior lateral side of the leg, 3 cun below ST-35 Dubi, one finger breadth (middle finger) from the anterior crest of the tibia (Figure 3.33).

Indications: Numbness, pain, and weakness on the lateral side of the crus.

GB-30 Huantiao

Location: On the buttock, at the junction of the middle third and lateral third of the line connecting the prominence of the great trochanter and the sacral hiatus, when the patient is in a lateral recumbent position with the thigh flexed (Figure 3.34).

Indications: Pain, numbness, and weakness in the lower limbs.

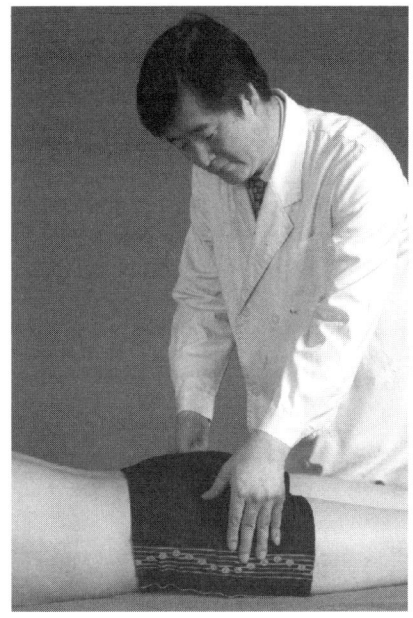

Figure 3.34 Digital pressing on GB-30 Huantiao

BL-54 Zhibian

Location: On the sacrum, level with the fourth posterior sacral foramen, 3 cun lateral to the median sacral crest (Figure 3.35).

Indications: Pain, numbness, and weakness in the lower limbs.

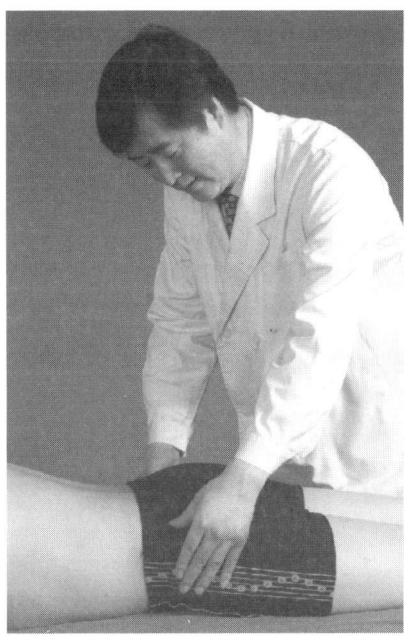

Figure 3.35 Digital pressing on BL-54 Zhibian

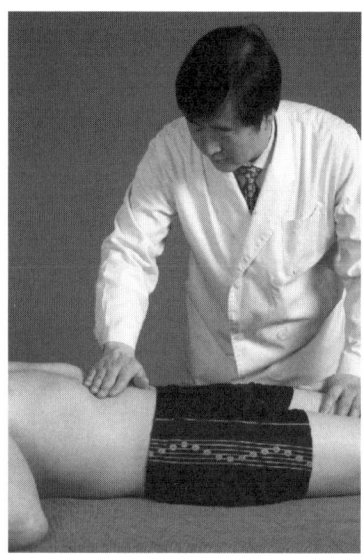

Also useful in treating cervical spondylotic myelopathy is the technique of rubbing the abdomen (see p.61).

Use the fingers for rubbing the chest, and the palms for rubbing on the abdomen. This will release qi in the chest and abdomen, and alleviate the symptoms in the chest and abdomen (Figure 3.36).

Figure 3.36 Rubbing the abdomen

SYMPATHETIC CERVICAL SPONDYLOSIS

Because the symptoms of sympathetic cervical spondylosis are relatively numerous, and the affected region is vast, the manipulations should be used according to the patient's symptoms. Digital pressing on acupoints and manipulations on local parts can be used.

For example, for heart-throb and precordial pain, digital pressing of PC-6 Neiguan, circular rubbing, and pushing outwards across the chest and precordium can be used.

BN-17 Danzhong

Location: On the anterior midline, level with the fourth intercostal space, at the midpoint of the line joining the nipples (Figure 3.37).

Indications: Oppression in the chest, being short of breath, palpitations.

For dysfunction of stomach and intestine, rubbing the abdomen (Figure 3.38), and digital pressing of acupoints on the abdomen can be used.

RN-12 Zhongwan

Location: On the anterior midline, 4 cun above the centre of the umbilicus (Figure 3.39).

Indications: Anorexia, abdominal distension, subnormal function of the stomach and intestine.

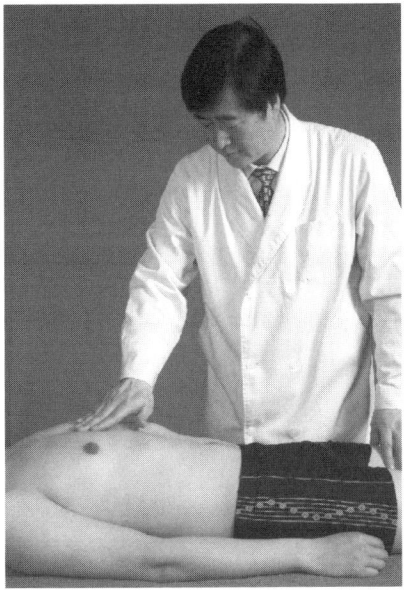 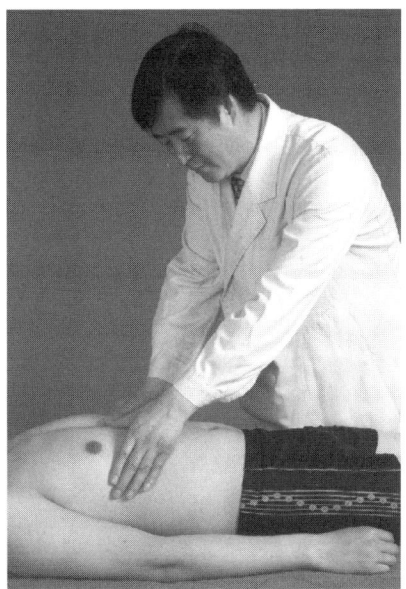

Figure 3.37 Manipulations for palpitations

a. Circular rubbing on Danzhong   *b. Pushing outwards across the chest*

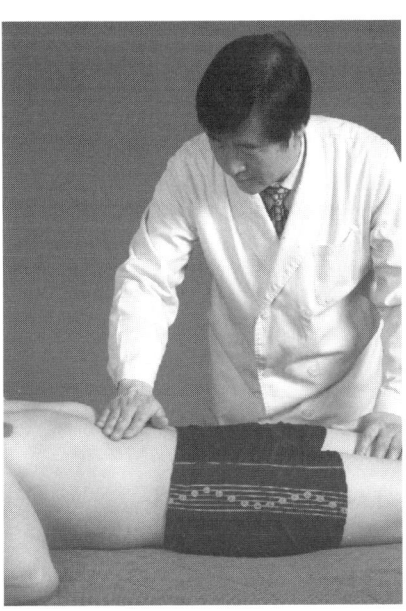 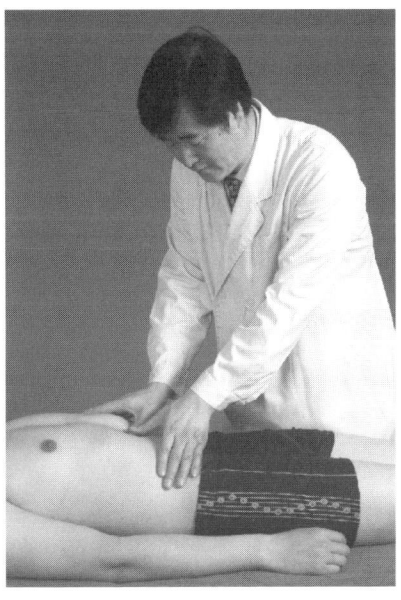

Figure 3.38 Rubbing abdomen   *Figure 3.39 Digital pressing on*
                                            RN-12 Zhongwan

4. Pulling manipulation for readjustment

For spinous process misalignment, that is, rotation around the vertical axis of a cervical vertebra, the technique of pulling the rotated and localized neck can be used (Figure 3.40). Make sure that the patient is relaxed when performing this manipulation. To relax muscle, manipulations can be used; to help the patient relax emotionally, use conversation and put patient into a relaxed posture.

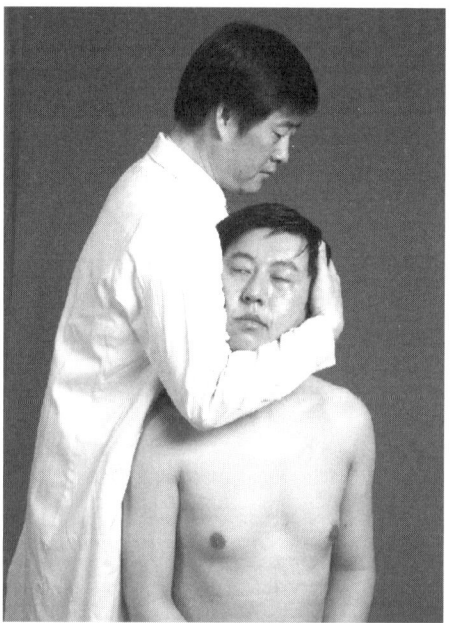

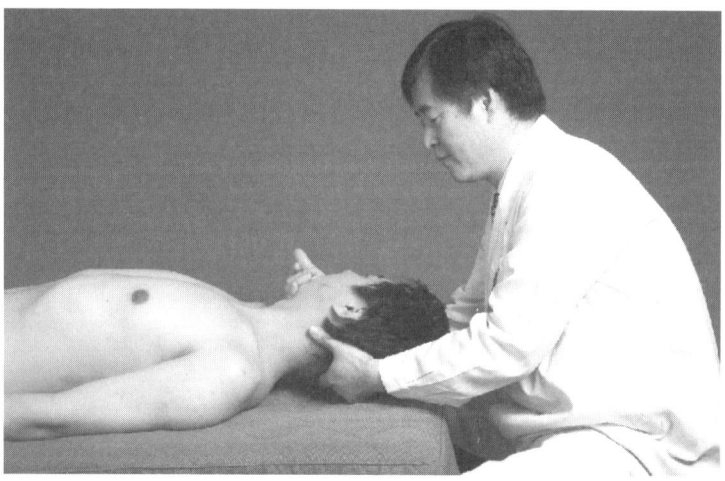

Figure 3.40 Pulling manipulation for readjustment

5. Traction for decompression

Use traction of the head and neck (Figure 3.41) to reduce the force of compression on an intervertebral disk, increase intervertebral space, enlarge the intervertebral foramen, decrease compression of nerves, the vertebral artery, and spinal cord, and restore injured tissue.

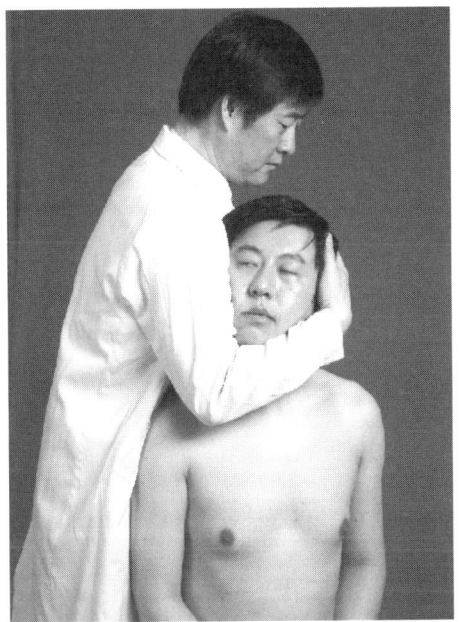
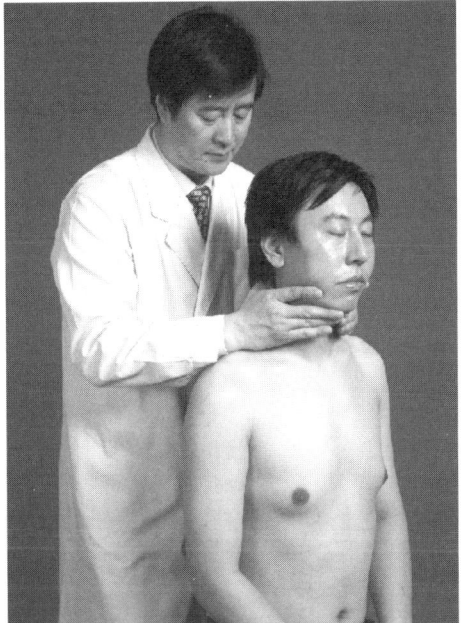
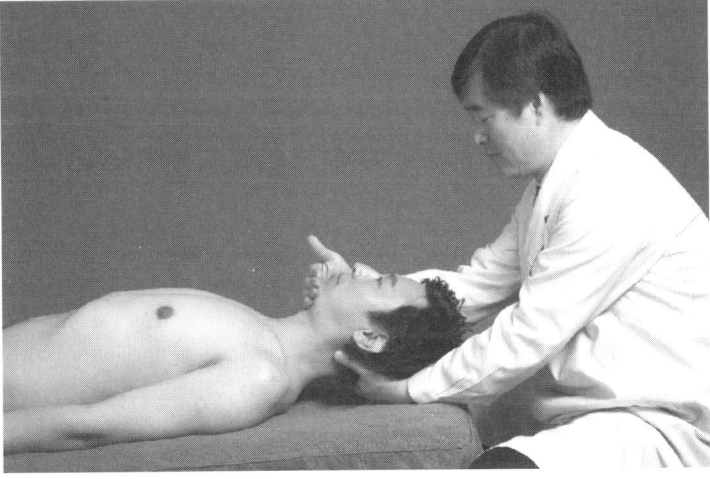

Figure 3.41 Traction for decompression

6. Rotation to improve the range of movement

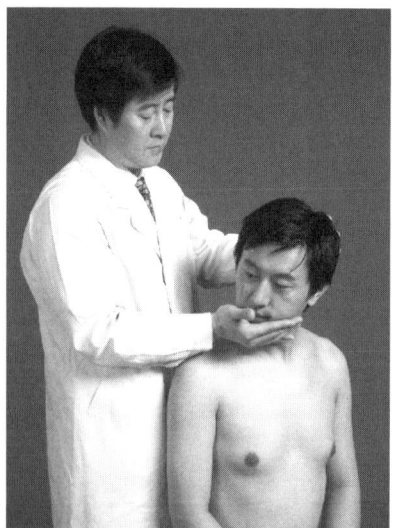

For restriction of movement in the nape, neck-rotating manipulation (Figure 3.42) can be used to restore normal function in the nape. It should be used with caution, otherwise dizziness may be exacerbated. This manipulation can be combined with traction of the head and neck.

Figure 3.42 Neck-rotating manipulation

7. Lateral pulling manipulation to improve the range of movement

For restricted movement of the nape in bending laterally, when pain is located on the opposite side, lateral pulling manipulation of the cervical spine should be performed (Figure 3.43). If the pain is located on the same side of the neck as the restricted movement, this technique is not advisable.

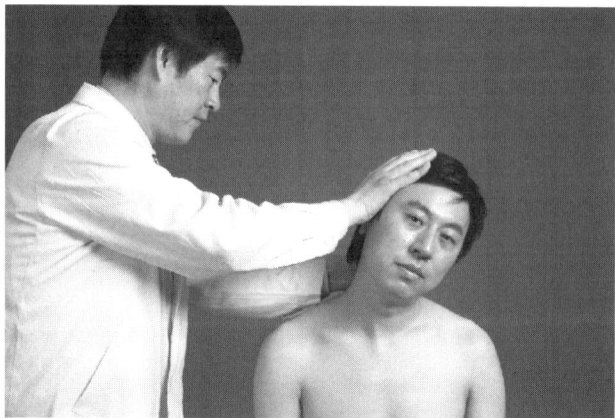

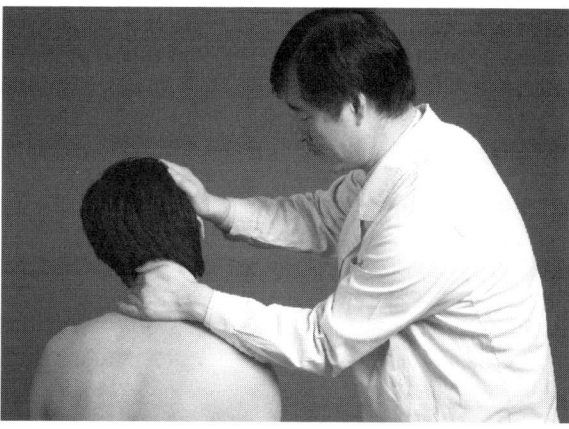

Figure 3.43 Lateral pulling manipulation to improve range of movement

8. Finishing manipulations

This series of manipulations consolidates the therapeutic effect of the preceding manipulations. They are used to relieve rigidity of muscles, activate collaterals, alleviate emergent pain, and finish the treatment. The following four manipulations are always used as finishing manipulations, and can be used according to the individual case.

Method 1: Pushing to dredge the meridian passage (Figure 3.44). Apply pushing manipulation to the Governor Vessel and the two lateral lines of the Bladder Meridian of Hand-Taiyang on the back: from the upper part to the lower part, from the upper back to the lower back, and then move quickly back to the upper back with the hand slightly attached to the skin, and start over again.

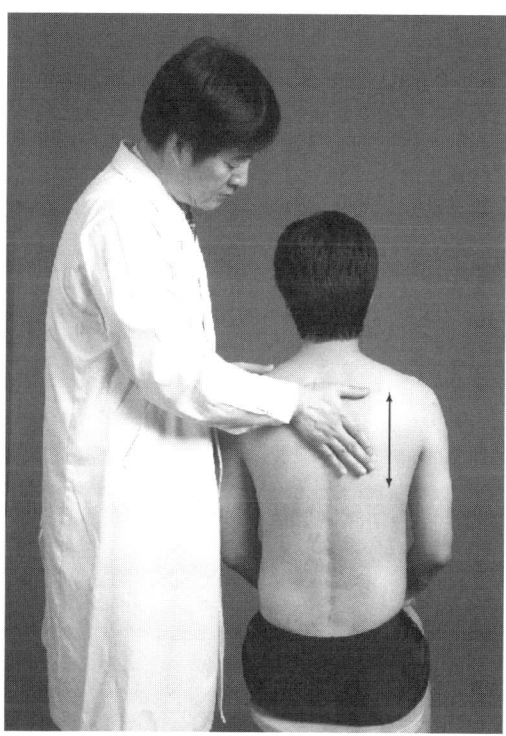

Figure 3.44 Pushing manipulation to dredge the meridian passage

Method 2: Rubbing to-and-fro for warming and dredging (Figure 3.45). Apply rubbing to-and-fro to the Small Intestine Meridian of Hand-Taiyang and the Sanjiao Meridian of Hand-Shaoyang on the shoulder. Thenar rubbing may also be done, with the forearm held perpendicular to the area to be treated.

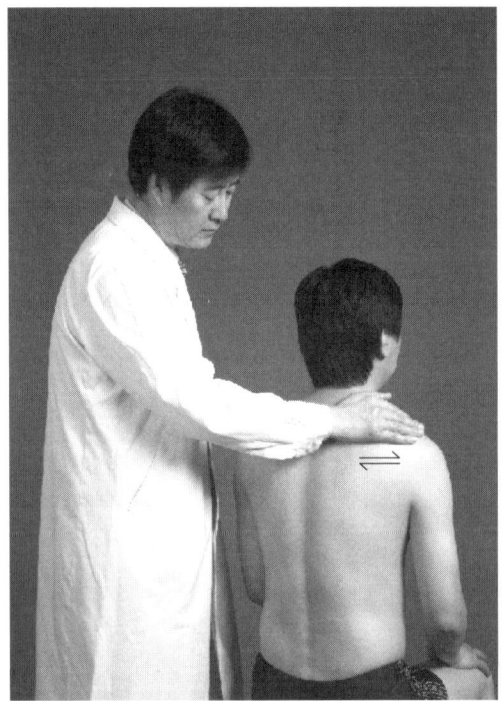 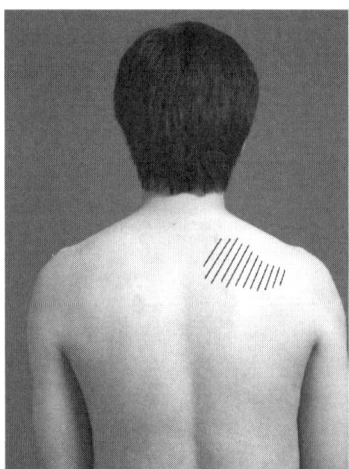

Figure 3.45 Rubbing to-and-fro for warming and dredging

Method 3: Laterally percussing for loosening tendons (Figure 3.46). Apply lateral percussing to the shoulder. This can be done with two hands alternately; or put the palms together and percuss with both hands. Lateral percussing should be done lightly on the nape and occiput.

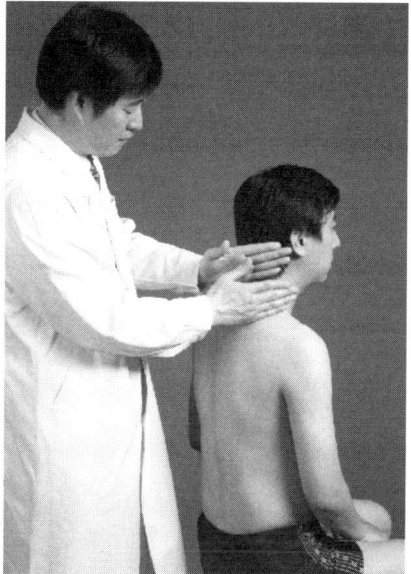

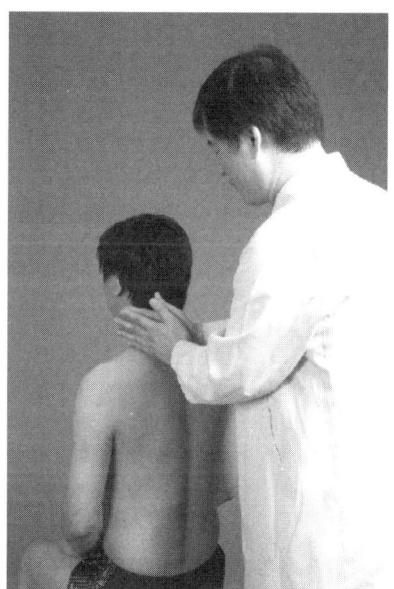
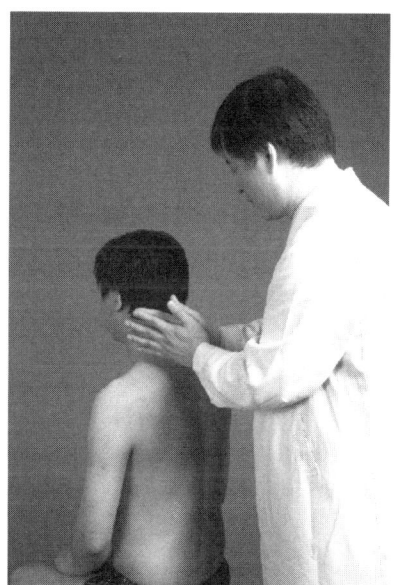

Figure 3.46 Laterally percussing for loosening tendons

Method 4: Grasping for loosening tendons (Figure 3.47). Apply grasping manipulation to relax the muscles of the shoulder. Make sure that the frequency of the manipulation is fast to begin with, and then becomes slower.

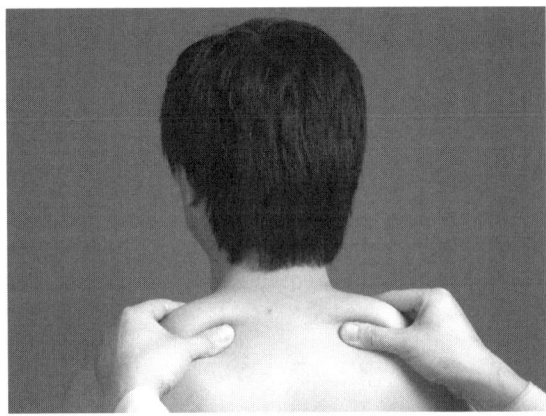

Figure 3.47 Grasping for loosening tendons

Section II Errors to Avoid in Massage Therapy Treatment

Performing massage therapy without a clear diagnosis

To perform any treatment without a clear diagnosis is strongly prohibited in all departments in clinics. There are occasional reports, for example, of shoulder pain, when numbness of the upper limb is caused by angina. An apex tumor of the lung has been misdiagnosed as cervical spondylotic radiculopathy, and one patient with acoustic neuroma and ophthalmic disease was misdiagnosed as having the vertebral artery type of cervical spondylosis. So treatment should be performed only after clarifying the diagnosis, and moreover special symptoms should be noted in order to reach a correct diagnosis. The diagnosis should be reviewed if the treatment is not successful.

Misapplication of pulling manipulation

Performing pulling manipulation on every patient, and doing it in such a way as to produce the sound of a click in the neck, disregarding the subluxation of cervical vertebrae or the patient's constitution, is a relatively ubiquitous problem. The reason why the patient finds some ease after pulling is that it stretches the muscles, and stretching the muscles can relax a patient – that's why the patient feels easy. Loosening a joint excessively has a negative effect on the joint's stability. A trade-off between loosening joints and temporarily relaxing muscles is false. The recommendation is to learn judgment according to the criteria for applying pulling manipulation, and use it with discretion.

Over-energetic Tuina

Over-energetic Tuina does harm to both the patient and the doctor. So an appropriate level of stimulus should be applied to treatment, such that 'a manipulation should cause the patient no suffering.'

Failure to consider local anatomy

If digital kneading or pushing manipulation with one finger are carried out with too much force on the upper cervical region, this can easily stimulate the vertebral artery, and cause fainting. So too strong a stimulus is inadvisable when performing manipulation on the upper cervical region, especially when treating patients with the vertebral artery type of cervical spondylosis.

Poor judgment

Pulling manipulation of the rotated and localized neck can easily stimulate the vertebral artery and spinal cord, and so it should be used with caution, or prohibited, when treating patients with the vertebral artery type of cervical spondylosis, or cervical spondylotic myelopathy, and especially those with lateral hyperplasia of the uncovertebral joint shown by X-ray, or herniated disk shown in a CT scan.

Chapter *4*

Prevention of Cervical Spondylosis

Section I Dos and Don'ts for the Neck

Choose your pillow with care

The height of the pillow is all-important for keeping the cervical spine healthy. A pillow that is either too high or too low is harmful for the cervical spine (Figure 4.1).

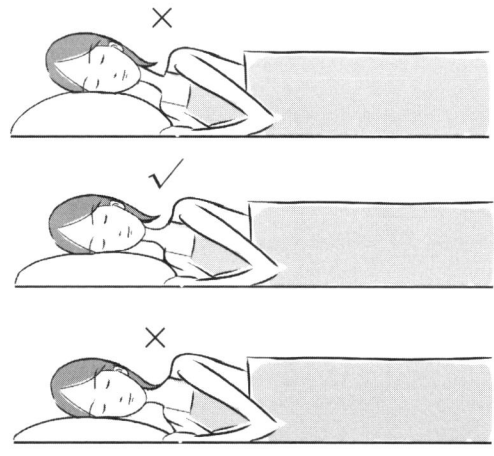

Figure 4.1 A pillow that is too high or too low is harmful for the neck

Most people get used to lying on their side when sleeping, so the height of the pillow needs to fill the space between the lateral side of the head and the lateral side of the shoulder, taking into account the consistency of the pillow and the consistency of the bed: the greater the distance between the lateral side of the head and the lateral side of the shoulder, the higher the pillow, relatively speaking. A soft pillow should be even thicker. A low pillow is appropriate for someone who is accustomed to lie on their back when sleeping.

Don't bend your neck forward for too long

When people bend their neck forward, the muscles of the nape tense, and with the passing of time, muscle strain sets in (Figure 4.2). Persistent strain leads to a change in the physiological curve of the nape, and in turn there is degeneration and hyperplasia of the cervical vertebrae. So drooping the head is a major cause of malfunction in the nape.

Long periods of bending down should be avoided as much as possible in daily life. If a person has to spend a long time at work slumped over a desk, he needs to have ten minutes' break once an hour, and to do some exercises of the nape in order to relax the muscles. This will also help increase efficiency at work and keep the eyes healthy.

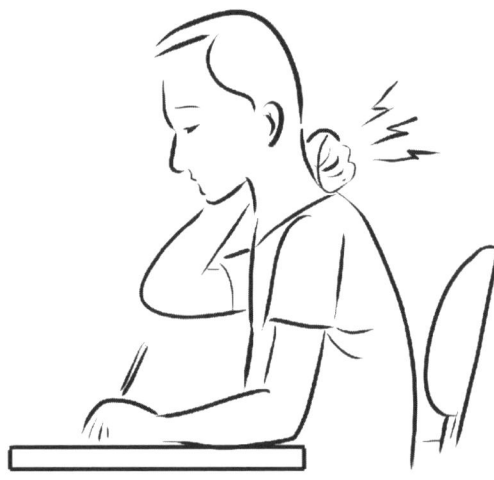

Figure 4.2 Tension and pain in the nape when drooping the head forwards

Avoid exposure to cold

A common cause of cervical spondylosis is exposure to cold. Exposure to cold, especially of the lateral part of the nape and the shoulder on one side of the body (for example, cold air from air conditioning on one side of the body), causes asymmetrical tension in the muscles on either side of the nape and shoulders, and triggers discomfort there (Figure 4.3). So the nape and shoulders should be protected from long, persistent cold stimuli, such as chilling from an air conditioner in summer, and you need to dress warmly enough, when going out in winter, to protect the nape from the cold.

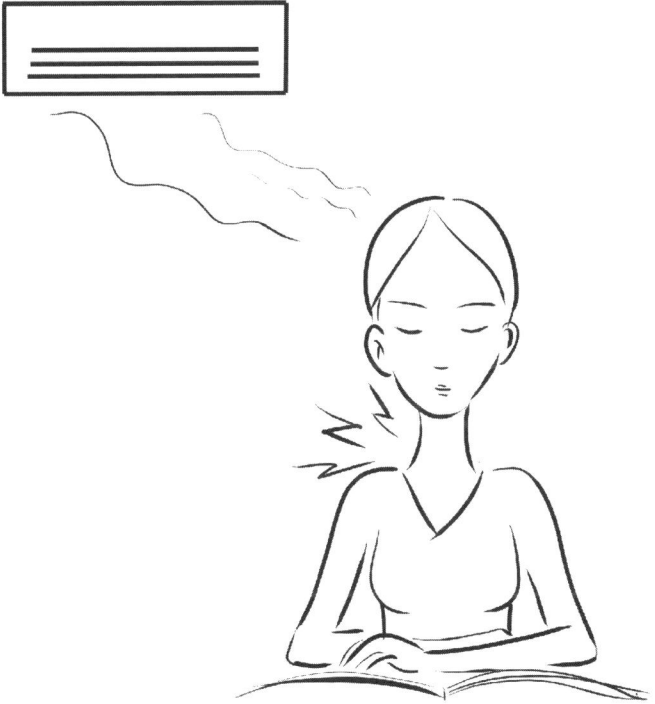

*Figure 4.3 Muscles on one side contract when the air conditioner
blows on that side of the nape*

Avoid dangerous working conditions

Those who have cervical spondylosis, especially the vertebral artery type of cervical spondylosis, should avoid working in hazardous conditions – for example, driving, installing and maintaining electrical equipment, working high above the ground, underwater jobs (Figure 4.4).

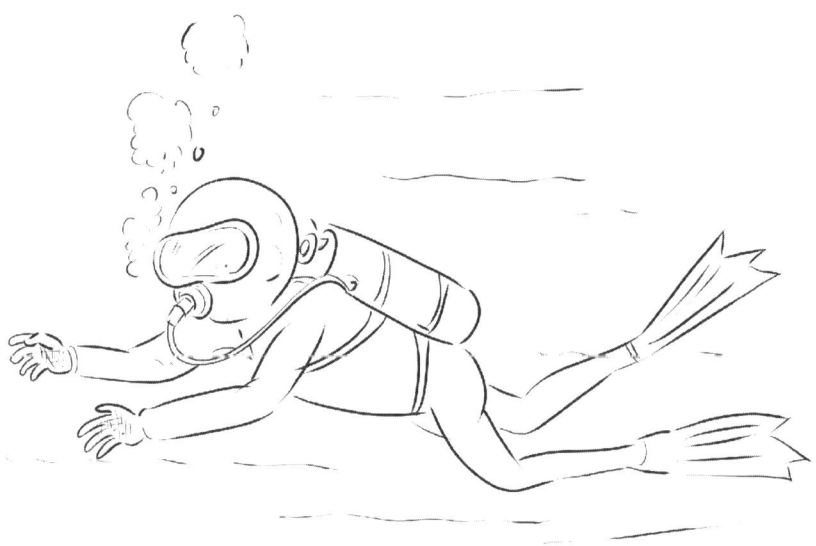

Figure 4.4 Dangerous jobs/situations

Care of the neck when using a computer

Computers bring people extreme convenience, but also some problems. Attention should be paid to the following in order to prevent the cervical spine from being harmed by overuse of the computer (Figure 4.5): don't overuse the computer; don't use it for too long at a time; adjust the angle of the monitor so as to let the head and neck relax. To put the monitor in the right position, we recommend that it be placed in front of the operator; if it has to be positioned to the left or the right side, it should be moved from one side to the other side at fixed intervals. Pay attention to the position of the keyboard and mouse.

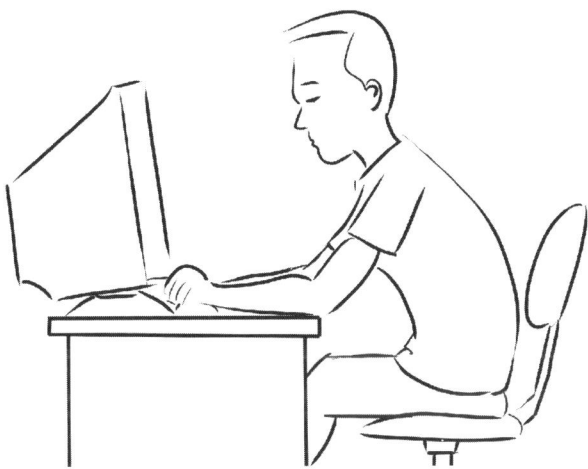

Figure 4.5 The cervical vertebrae are harmed by sitting badly when using a computer

Section II Self-Massage for the Neck

Squeezing and pressing the muscles on both sides of the nape

Manipulation: Relax and sit on the stool; put one hand behind the neck, and exert force from both sides of the nape towards the center with the palms and heels of the hands, in order to relax the muscles of the nape. The manipulation is applied to the nape from the top downward. Repeat ten times (Figure 4.6). Squeezing and pressing can also be combined with kneading.

Key point: The force should be deep and firm.

Function: Relieve muscle spasm in the nape; prevent and cure disorders such as muscle strain in the nape and shoulders, cervical spondylosis, and stiff neck. This is important for those doing long-term desk work.

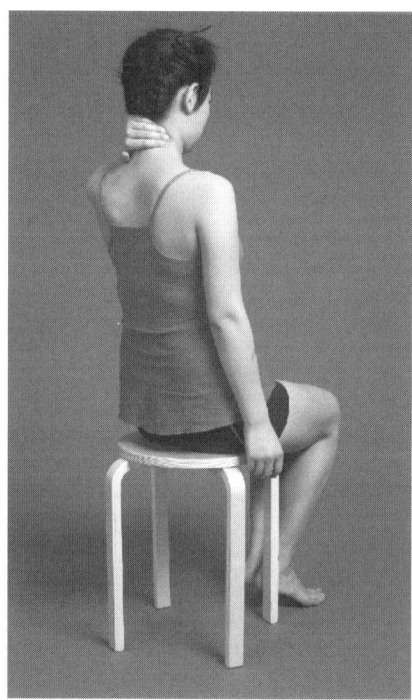

Figure 4.6 Squeezing and pressing the muscles on both sides of the nape

Pressing and kneading the muscles with four fingers on both sides of the nape

Manipulation: Relax and sit on the stool; put the four fingers of both hands behind the neck, and knead the muscles on both sides of the nape in circles with the fingers, so as to relax the muscles of the nape. The manipulation is applied to the nape from the top downwards. Repeat ten times (Figure 4.7).

Key point: The force should be deep and firm.

Function: Relieve muscle spasm in the nape, prevent and cure disorders such as muscle strain in the nape and shoulders, cervical spondylosis, and stiff neck. It is important for those doing long-term desk work.

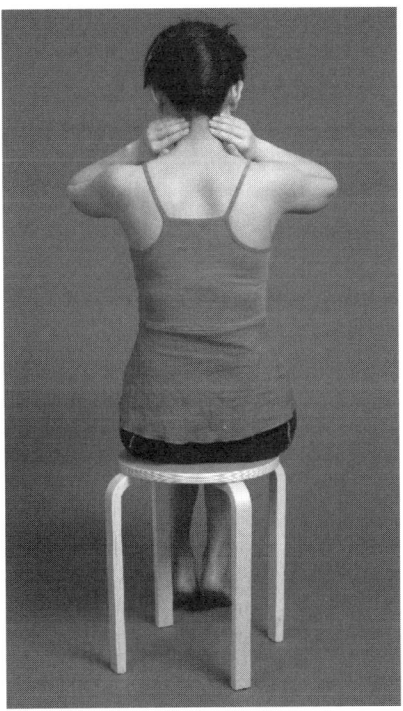

Figure 4.7 Pressing and kneading
muscles with four fingers on both
sides of the nape

Digital pressing and kneading on acupoints of the occiput

Manipulation: Digital pressing and kneading of acupoints such as GB-20 Fengchi (Figure 4.8), BL-10 Tianzhu, SJ-17 Yifeng, with index fingers and middle fingers of both hands.

Key point: In digital pressing and kneading of GB-20 Fengchi, the force should first be applied perpendicularly to the skin, and then medially and superiorly. Optimal force will produce an aching feeling in the area that is being treated. When digital pressing and kneading BL-10 Tianzhu, and SJ-17 Yifeng, it is fine if the force is perpendicular to the skin.

Function: Relax the muscles on both sides of the nape; cure symptoms in the head, such as headache and dizziness. It can also be used to help blurred vision, and cure diseases of the eyes.

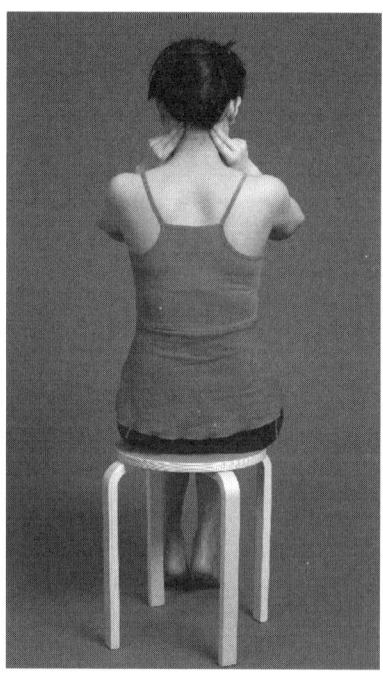

*Figure 4.8 Digital pressure and
kneading of GB-20 Fengchi*

Pinching and grasping the shoulders

Manipulation: Pinch and grasp the muscles of both shoulders alternately (Figure 4.9).

Key point: When pinching and grasping, the force can be gentle at first, then exert more force and combine pinching and grasping with slight lifting. Finally, relax. Repeat until there is aching and distending, and a warm, comfortable feeling.

Function: Relax the muscles of the nape and shoulders; remove the feeling of fatigue in the nape; cure diseases of the nape and shoulders.

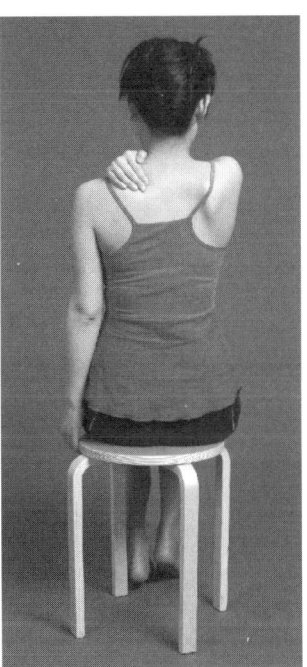 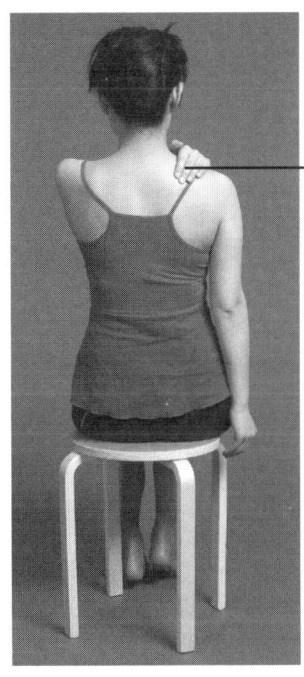

Pinch and lift until there is a distending soreness in the area of the shoulders

Figure 4.9 Pinching and grasping the shoulders

Gently patting the nape and shoulders

Manipulation: Make hollow fists with both hands, and gently pat the nape and shoulders with the fists (Figure 4.10).

Key point: Use the left hand to pat the right side, and the right hand to pat the left side. Don't exert too much force when patting; the patting will be right if there is a feeling of relaxation and comfort.

Function: Relax the muscles of nape and shoulders.

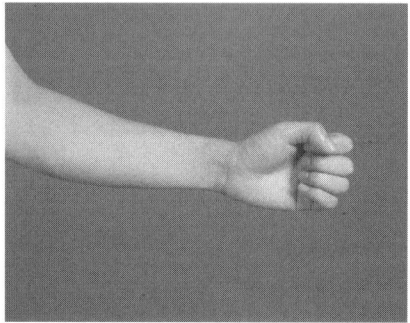

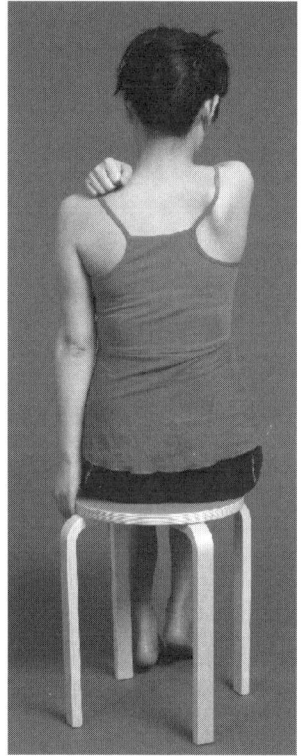
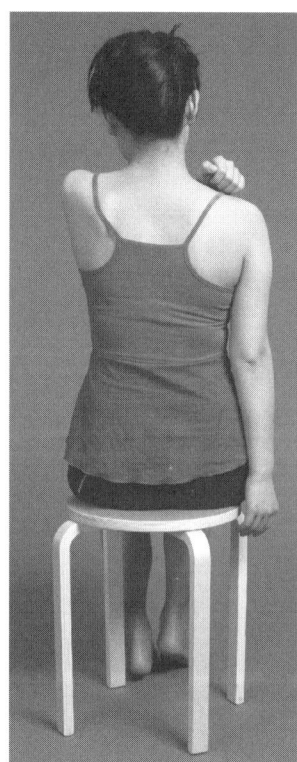

Figure 4.10 Gently patting the nape and shoulders

Section III Functional Exercises for the Neck

Forwards bending and backwards bending

Take a seated or standing position while doing this exercise. First, push the head upwards, and then bend the neck forwards and backwards (Figure 4.11). This exercise is used to improve the range of movement when there's restriction of movement in bending forwards, backwards, and laterally. Keep both eyes open when doing the exercise; speed should be slow; hold the posture for a while when bending forwards and backwards to the maximum extent. Bend forwards and backwards alternately. This technique is used to restore the function of bending forwards and backwards.

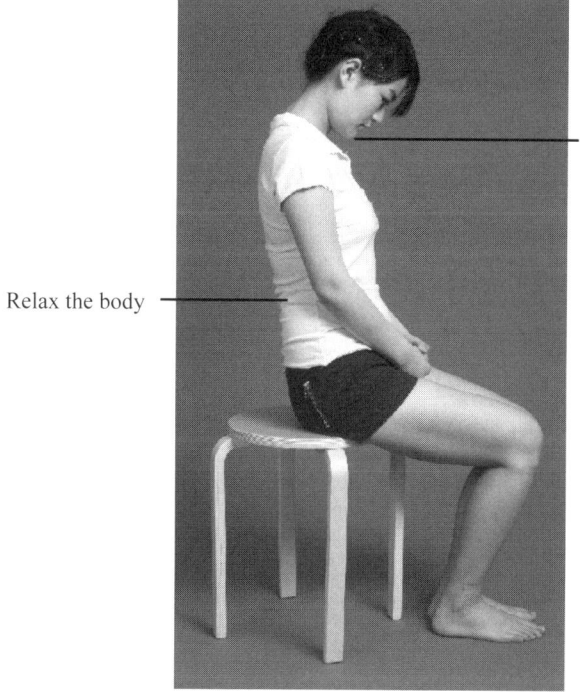

Bend forwards to the maximum extent

Relax the body

a

Figure 4.11 Bending forwards and backwards

Bend backwards to
the maximum extent

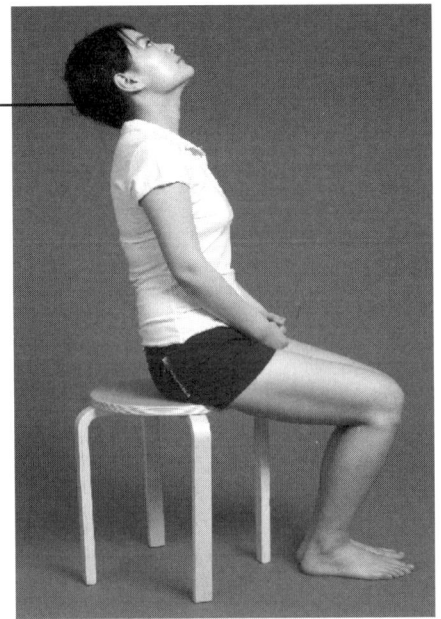

b

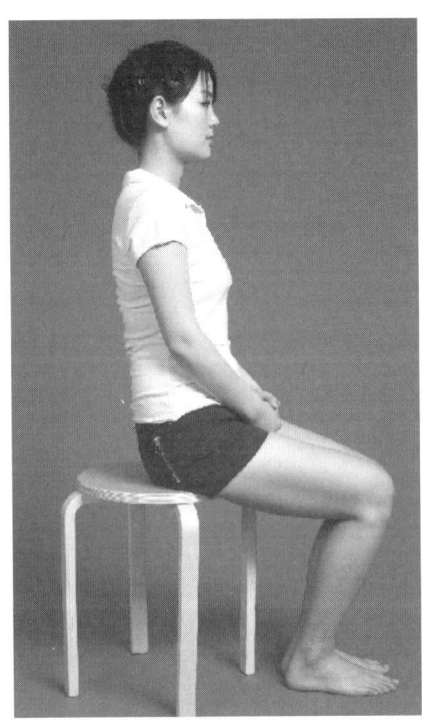

c

Lateral bending

Take a seated or standing position while doing this exercise. First, push the head upwards, and then bend the neck laterally (Figure 4.12). Keep both eyes open when doing the exercise; speed should be low; hold the posture for a while. Bend laterally to the maximum extent. This technique is used to restore the function of lateral bending.

Bend laterally to the maximum extent

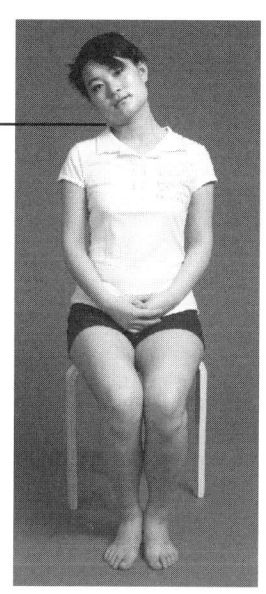

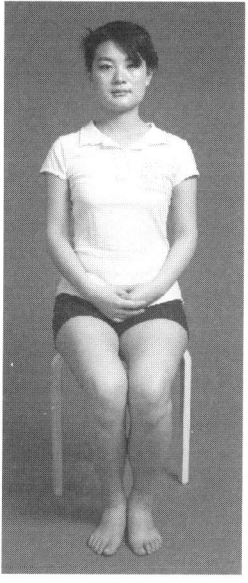 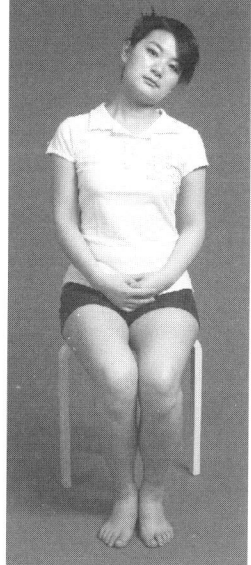

Figure 4.12 Lateral bending

Turning

Take a sitting or standing position while doing this exercise. Stand with arms akimbo; turn the head to one side; when turned to the maximum extent (Figure 4.13), hold the posture for a while, and then turn to the other side. This technique is used to restore the function of turning.

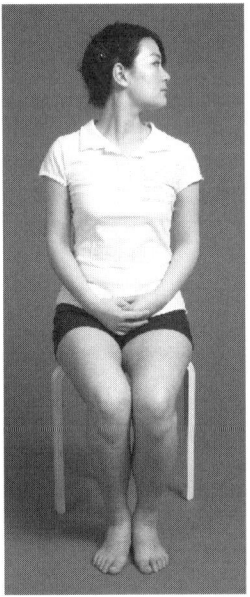

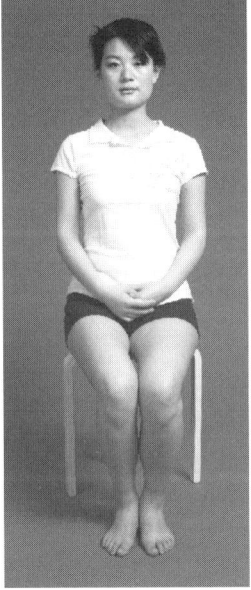 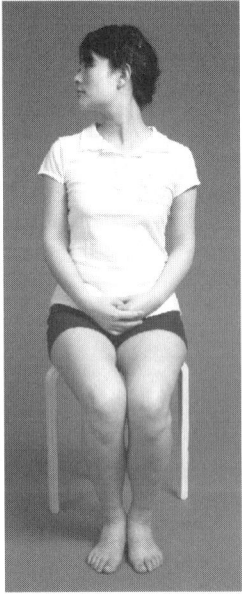

Figure 4.13 Turning

Antagonistic training

Take a sitting or standing position while doing this exercise. With the hands laced behind the neck, exert gentle force forwards with both hands while bending the neck backward. The force exerted by the hands opposes the force created by bending the neck backwards (Figure 4.14 and 4.15). Hold for five seconds, and rest for five seconds; then, with the hands laced on the forehead, exert gentle force backwards with both hands while bending the neck forwards. The force exerted by the hands opposes the force created by bending the neck forwards. Hold for five seconds, and rest for five seconds. This technique is used to relax the muscles on the anterior and posterior side of neck, nape, and shoulder, and to increase the strength of the muscles of the neck and shoulder.

Head leaned back
Exert force forward
with both hands

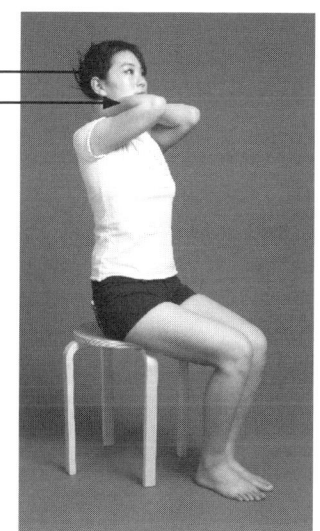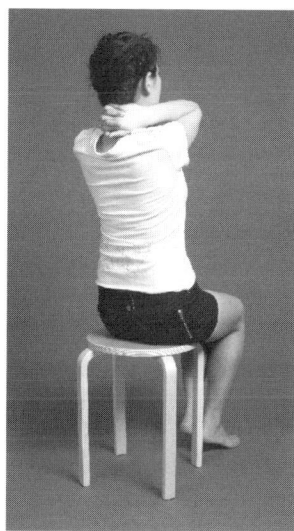

Figure 4.14 Antagonistic training (1)

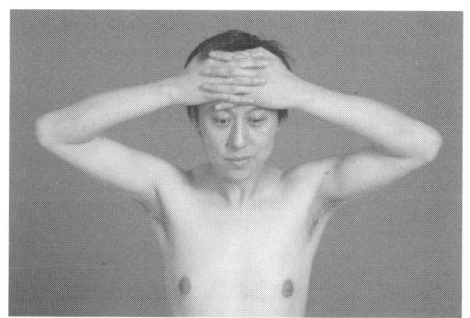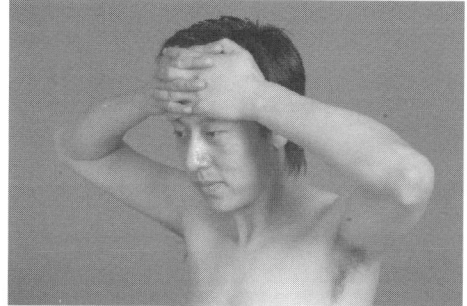

Figure 4.15 Antagonistic training (2)

Throwing out the chest

Take a seated or standing position while doing this exercise. Throw out the chest and look up, then push both shoulders backwards, vigourously (Figure 4.15). Hold the posture for five seconds, rest for five seconds, then relax. This technique is used to relax the muscles of the shoulders and back.

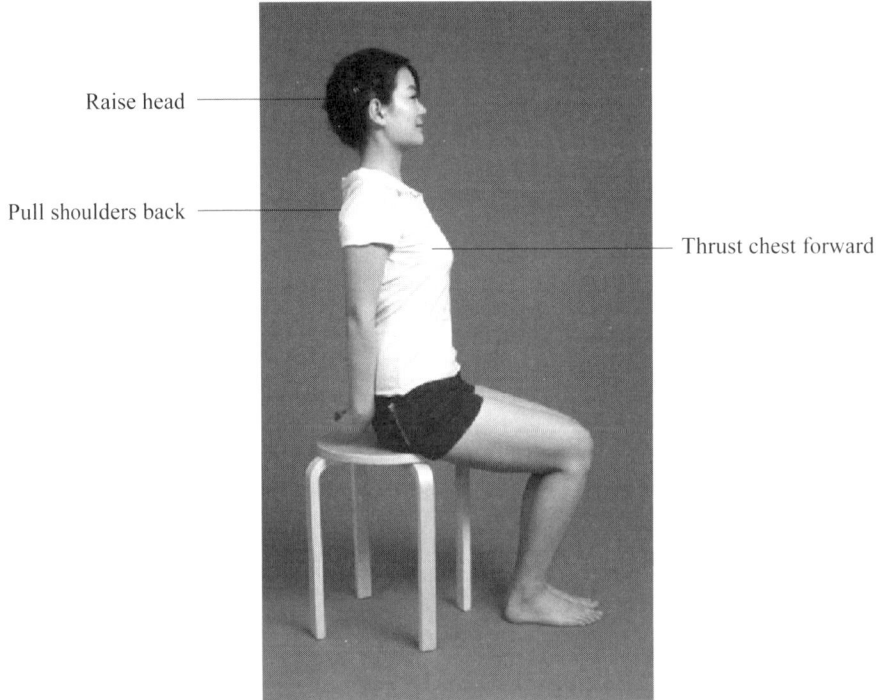

Raise head

Pull shoulders back

Thrust chest forward

Figure 4.16 Throwing out the chest

At the beginning stage, do the five exercises mentioned above 2–5 times a day; each time repeat every exercise ten times. If there is no discomfort, the exercises can be done more often.